P9-BZQ-243

The SNACK FACTOR Diet

The SNACK FACTOR Diet

The Secret to Losing Weight—
by Eating MORE

KERI GLASSMAN, M.S., R.D.
with Sarah Mahoney

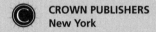

CROWN PUBLISHERS
New York

Copyright © 2007 by Keri Glassman

All rights reserved.
Published in the United States by Crown Publishers, an imprint of the
Crown Publishing Group, a division of Random House, Inc., New York.
www.crownpublishing.com

Crown is a trademark and the Crown colophon is a registered trademark of
Random House, Inc.

Library of Congress Cataloging-in-Publication Data

Glassman, Keri.
The snack factor diet : the secret to losing weight—by eating more / Keri Glassman.
— 1st ed.
p.   cm.
1. Weight loss—Psychological aspects.   2. Energy metabolism.   3. Reducing
diets—Recipes.   4. Snack foods.   I. Title.

RM222.2.G5377 2007
613.2'5—dc22

2006034844

ISBN 978-0-307-35147-0

Printed in the United States of America

Design by Helene Berinsky

10 9 8 7 6 5 4 3 2 1

First Edition

To my family:
Brett, Rex, and Maizy

ACKNOWLEDGMENTS

I could never thank all of the special people who have contributed to helping me write this book. The pages aren't long enough. . . . You all know who you are—thank you to my incredible extended family and friends.

A very special thanks to Julie Merberg for her vision for this book, her brilliance, and her patience. Without Julie's drive and passion, this book would still be inside of me. Julie helped me at every step and held my hand through this entire process. You are the very best!!

I'd like to thank Heather Jackson (and the team at Crown) for seeing the value of this book. You "got it" from the very beginning, and I appreciate your support.

Thank you to my two incredible associates Lara Englebardt Metz and Margaret Levy for being incredibly loyal employees, and for your hard work, devotion, and commitment to this project. The field of nutrition is lucky to have the two of you. This book would not have happened without you.

To Sarah Mahoney, who understood this book from the beginning and was simply a pleasure to work with. Thank you for "hearing" and "translating" me. You are wonderful!

Thank you to my clients, who have inspired me to be a better nutritionist and have helped me formulate this book so others can enjoy and learn from it. I take great pleasure in seeing you become healthier people.

A special thank-you to my incredible parents for their support of my education, career, goals, and dreams.

Most of all, thank you to my husband, Brett, for your unconditional support and love, and for reminding me of what is most important. And to my children, Rex and Maizy, who inspire me daily. Your smiles make every day a good day.

CONTENTS

Introduction

Eat Up! It's Healthy

"I know what to do; I just don't know how to do it!" This is what nearly all of my clients tell me during our first meeting. And these days, it's true—there is no shortage of information about how to eat a healthy, well-balanced diet. In fact, when it comes to food, my typical client is incredibly smart. He or she has usually read dozens of books and magazine articles on health and nutrition, spent hours examining the ingredient labels on the food he or she consumes, and agonized over what counts as a "good" or "bad" fat. She's had more conversations about carbs than most people have had about politics, religion, or where to go on their next vacation. What's more, my average client has tried—and usually given up on—upward of five diets!

And I don't just mean formal diets from the bestseller lists, from grapefruit to cabbage to all-protein to blood type. (Trust me, I've seen refugees from every diet known to man.) These busy, on-the-go people, who are usually very happy and successful in most areas of their lives, have poured amazing amounts of time and energy into developing their personal eating systems, too. You probably know the kinds of eating plans I mean: "I'll only eat pretzels." Or "I'll be good all week, and eat what I want on weekends." Or "I'll be good all day, and then splurge at dinner." Or when imagination fails them and they completely run out of ideas, they vow to not eat *anything.* Then they wonder why they collapse in a frazzled heap in front of the office vending machine at 4:00 P.M., and find themselves tearing through a bag of Doritos.

The belief that we'll finally hit on the perfect diet just for us is why dieting has become a multibillion-dollar industry. But if there's one thing I think all of us can agree on, it is that those plans just aren't working. That's why people hire me to help them change the way they eat and why you're looking at this book right now. Chances are, just like my clients when they first come to see me, you want to lose weight and haven't been able to do it on your own. And chances are, you're more than a little ticked off about it. But please understand that you're not alone: *60 percent of America is overweight.* Now, go back and reread that last sentence. I know it's a statistic you've already heard a million times. But what that 60 percent means is that, even though we're armed with all this great information about nutrition, being overweight is more common than being healthy. Put another way, only four out of ten American adults are able to control their weight.

So what makes all these smart people—who are so successful in other ways—fail? When I take a look at my clients' diets, I notice two major errors, both part of a common theme that I believe is undermining America's effort to get back into its "thin" jeans. Despite all their knowledge about dieting, they're lousy snackers. They are making two mistakes:

1. Snacking poorly. Maybe they choose seemingly harmless foods, such as pretzels or granola, which turn out to deliver plenty of empty calories and leave them hungry again before they know it. Or they eat junk food—stuff they know is bad for them but is easy and available. And these poor snack choices don't just affect their weight and caloric intake. They contribute to fluctuating blood sugar and crashing energy levels, all of which set people up to make self-defeating food choices the next chance they get.

And beyond the day-to-day damage of poor snacking, there are long-term health consequences, including heart disease. OK, I know it may sound pretty doom-and-gloom of me to say that your 3:00 P.M. M&M habit is affecting your life expectancy, but it's true. After all, it's the little habits we have that add up to our overall health picture and contribute to future heart disease! And it is the small changes you make daily that have the most profound effects.

2. Not snacking at all. By not snacking—even though it may make them feel virtuous—they are disrupting their blood sugar levels, which almost always results in overeating at their next meal. This, in turn, affects their weight (which goes up) and energy level (which goes down). They end up eating whatever is available first, which often means nutritionally bankrupt food choices. (Anyone who's ever consumed double helpings of a food he or she doesn't even like knows exactly what I mean!) And what's worse, because overeating feels so normal, these people often blunt their awareness of the number-one weight-loss tool *all* of us have: the ability to recognize when we're no longer hungry and stop eating.

THE RIGHT SNACKS ARE JUST RIGHT

Wait a minute, you're thinking, *So, snacking is not good and not snacking is not good?* No! *The Snack Factor Diet* will show you how the right snacks—nutrient-dense foods, eaten at the right times of day—will *anchor your health*, steady your mood, and make weight loss as easy as possible. That's what this book is all about—changing the way you think of the word *snack*. Right now, to you, *snack* probably means a tasty extra, something "good" dieters should do without, even if it is only a 100-calorie pack!

And who could blame you for misunderstanding the word? After all, the snack food industry is a multibillion-dollar industry; Americans spend about $6 billion a year on potato chips alone and $37 billion on soft drinks! For most of us, snack foods have been guilty pleasures, whether our tastes run to salty foods (chips and pretzels) or to sweets (cookies and candy). Either way, we've gotten used to thinking of them as plain old calories, and we don't expect anything more from them than a false sense of fullness that will maybe last us to the next meal, when we'll eat *real* food.

Not only are the foods most of us think of as snack foods terrible food choices (don't worry—I'm going to teach you that snacks are real food, too, and introduce you to hundreds of delicious, wholesome, and easy snacks in Chapter 5), but we've fallen in love with eating them in an unhealthy way. Sometimes, we get tricked by packaging, like those 100-calorie bags of cookies. My clients confess that most of the time they're gobbling these extra calories mindlessly, while they're on the move or doing something else. Eating is done without much consciousness, nibbling as they answer e-mails, drive to pick up the kids, or wait to get their hair colored. It seems as if there's never any time to think about what we are putting in our bodies, let alone why we are putting it there. I am here to help you with that!

I teach my clients that to get to the weight they want—and into the clothes they love—they need to do what this country likes best, and that's snack. But we need to snack smarter. By the time you've finished reading this book, the word *snack* will have taken on an entirely new meaning. Smart snacking will become your secret weapon and your passport to the weight you want to be. Within just three days, the Snack Factor Diet will help you

- Lose weight
- Improve energy
- Stabilize blood sugar levels—no more mood swings throughout the day!
- Prevent constipation (keep you "regular")

And that's just for starters. Before you finish this four-week plan, you'll have made real progress in meeting longer-term goals, as well. You will have started to

- Prevent heart disease, diabetes, and some cancers
- Improve your skin
- Protect against aging
- Sharpen your mental skills
- Get happy—literally!

At this point, my clients generally roll their eyes and think, "She *must* be exaggerating." But I'm not. As a registered dietician who's devoted years of my life to understanding the science behind snacking, I can tell you that snacking is truly the Holy Grail of nutrition, with plenty of solid science behind it. Much of the evidence boils down to the power of *satiety*, a buzzword that will change your diet destiny forever. Simply put, it means how satisfied (or "satiated") you feel by any given food.

Remember the last time you ate a handful of jellybeans and how quickly you devoured 150 calories worth? (That's only about thirty-seven of those minuscule Jelly Belly beans!) Was your craving satisfied? Or did you dive back into the bag, again and again, for just one more handful? Now, remember the last time you ate some peanut butter? Sure, you knew it was high in calories. But one spoonful on your toast was probably enough to keep you going all morning.

Chalk up the difference to satiety and get ready because *The Snack Factor Diet* is going to turn you on to literally hundreds of snack possibilities that will leave you so satisfied that you can get back to living your life and quit worrying about what you'll eat at your next meal.

THE SCIENCE BEHIND *THE SNACK FACTOR DIET*

It's as simple as this: snacking properly improves satiety. A study from a medical school in South Africa measured it this way: One group of healthy men ate breakfast in a single meal, while another group was given the same identical meal, but at intervals throughout the morning. When both groups sat down to lunch, the snackers weren't as hungry and ate smaller lunches than the big-breakfast group. And even better, they felt just as satisfied as if they had eaten a high-calorie lunch. Another study tracked a group of French adults and found that they ate, on average, 2.7 meals and 1.3 snacks each day. The satiety ratio was higher for snacks than for meals, and snacks consumed in the afternoon were found to be especially satisfying.

Much of the groundbreaking research on snacking, and

how eating frequency affects not just satiety but also metabolism, comes from France, where many people customarily eat a fourth meal each day, usually in the afternoon. Studies found that when regular fourth-meal eaters gave up that afternoon snack, they gained weight because they overate at other meals. And those who continued to eat four meals a day had a better metabolic profile, with a reduction in the secretion of insulin, an improvement in insulin resistance, and better blood glucose control.

Of course, those changes to the metabolic profile are huge for someone struggling to control diabetes (which unfortunately, thanks to our weight struggles, includes more Americans every day). But how eating frequency affects our insulin levels concerns anyone trying to manage his or her weight. And while certainly not all nutrition experts agree on this, many feel that the spiking and plunging insulin levels that come from sporadic eating affect mood and can make us irritable, tense, depressed, and even shaky.

Snacking—by getting people away from the self-defeating habits of starving and then stuffing themselves—also seems to shrink people's stomachs. One study tracked obese people on a very low-calorie diet for four weeks, and researchers found a reduction in stomach size that ranged from 27 to 36 percent. So it makes sense that people who eat smaller, more frequent, meals will begin to feel more satisfied with less food over time. (We'll get into food timing more in Chapter 1.)

Some people are lucky enough to develop this smart-snacking skill without thinking about it. A study of more than 3,200 men and women, conducted by Arizona State University, found that "multiple snackers"—people who naturally snack throughout the day when they are hungry, as I suggest my clients do—might just be inherently smarter about their food choices. These snackers made more prudent decisions about how much protein, cholesterol, calcium, and sodium they consumed each day, compared to people who never snacked or people who snacked only at one time each day (as during late-night *Seinfeld* reruns).

Research has also confirmed how snacking helps heart health. One clinical trial, for example, compared two groups of people eating the same diet. The first group ate six meals a day; the second group had the same foods in equal amounts, but they were served in irregular patterns, anywhere from three to nine meals a day. The results were impressive: smaller, more frequent meals resulted in lower LDL-cholesterol (a.k.a. the bad stuff), by reducing cholesterol synthesis in the liver. Total cholesterol fell 9 percent and LDL fell 14 percent. French studies have also shown that more frequent eaters have better lipid profiles.

THE BUSY PERSON'S DIET

There's another big scientific benefit from the Snack Factor Diet: it helps really busy people—the kind who tend to eat sporadically because of demanding jobs and crazy schedules—get into a regular eating routine. Research has demonstrated that for people trying to lose weight, the kind of routine eating that will become second nature on the Snack Factor Diet makes it easier to consume fewer calories, burn more calories after you eat, and promote steadier insulin levels; that means no more of those mood swings that so often come along with frantic I'll-just-grab-a-bite-on-the-way-to-my-next-appointment days.

I'm going to repeat that because it's such good news. The Snack Factor Diet will become second nature. Because this book will coach you not just on what to eat but also on the behavioral changes that go along with effective snacking, you'll be more likely to keep the weight off once you've lost it.

Best of all, snacking makes us happier. Researchers at the University of Wales divided a group of 150 women into three groups: one got no breakfast, one got a small breakfast (with 10 grams of carbs), and one got a larger meal (50 grams of carbs). After an hour and half, half of each breakfast-eating group also got a snack. Not only did the snack group report being in a better mood (and isn't that enough of a reason to start snacking, right now?), they were also sharper mentally and did better on a word-recall task that researchers gave them.

The point is that as long as we do not consume more calories (energy) than we use up, and we only eat when we are hungry (monitor your Hunger Quotient, or HQ), it's useful to split our total energy intake into as many nutrient-dense meals (designed to provide satiety) as our busy lives allow. And that's exactly what *The Snack Factor Diet* will teach you how to do.

WHAT'S AHEAD

In the next chapters, you will learn how to

- Monitor your *HQ* so that you know exactly when you need to eat
- Eat foods in the right *proportion* (protein, carbs, and fat)
- Choose *nutrient-dense* food for your snacks and meals to get the most out of the portions you eat
- Eat the right amount—*portions*—of these nutrient-dense foods to keep you supersatisfied, but not stuffed

Then in Chapter 5, you'll be guided through the Snack Factor Diet, which begins with a three-day "deprogramming" (of bad diet habits). You'll be able to construct your own meals and snacks from hundreds of choices, or you can follow the menus that I provide for you.

And when all is read and done, you will change the way you eat—forever!

What's Your HQ?

Using Your Hunger Quotient to Time Your Meals and Snacks

In our first session together, I always ask new clients, "How hungry are you when you eat?" Some people say they are never hungry. "How could I be? I'm always eating," they'll joke. Or they'll say, "Famished! I make myself wait to eat until I am starving, but I'm usually stuffed when I am done with a meal!" As basic as it is, many people—especially superbusy people—have a pretty feeble grasp of their Hunger Quotient. Maybe they just eat constantly, without thinking about it. Or they eat in such a spartan way—as if their virtue is measured by how few calories they consume—that they're never really satisfied. So when hunger does catch up with them, the pangs are powerful enough to knock them right into the nearest Taco Bell.

Years of not-so-great eating habits have made us tone-deaf to our body's hunger messages. Sure, we can listen to our body when it tells us we're tired, that we're coming down with a cold, or we've worked out too hard at the gym. But it's difficult for many of my clients—even the ones who know the exchange rate for the Japanese yen or the exact floor plan of Neiman Marcus—to answer this simple question: "Right now, how hungry am I?"

That's because most of us eat whether we are hungry or not. We eat because we think it's time to eat, or because the food tastes good, or maybe just because it's in front of us. The Snack Factor Diet will boost your HQ so that hunger—and only hunger—dictates your eating behavior.

Your hunger will tell you when it's time to eat your meals and snacks. You don't need to plan them around my schedule, or one devised by nutrition researchers in a lab somewhere. The whole point of the Snack Factor Diet is to help you find a regular eating pattern that suits your body, your metabolism, your goals, and your lifestyle. No matter what anyone tells you, there is no ideal time between meals. Everyone is unique and needs to know his or her HQ before picking up a fork.

Some people need to eat every few hours, while others should wait closer to four hours before eating between meals and snacks. I've got clients who are breakfast-snack-lunch-snack-dinner people, and I admit that's the style of eating that suits me best, too. But I've also got breakfast-lunch-snack-snack-dinner clients, and even a few breakfast-lunch-snack-snack-snack people! In fact, just by jotting down their HQ levels, my clients usually figure out their style in a few days.

THE EXCEPTION TO THE RULE

There is one exception to my let-your-hunger-be-your-guide rule, and that's breakfast. People are hungry at breakfast, even if they don't know it. Your body has probably gone ten to twelve hours with no nourishment at all, so it's running on empty. And the start of your workday—especially if it involves getting kids ready for school, fighting morning traffic, or diving into a less-than-scintillating sales report—often demands serious mental energy. In a perfect world, we would all wake up craving nutritious breakfasts that complemented our busy days.

The bad news is that many of my clients come to me with the reverse metabolic scenario: they skip breakfast, or if they eat at all, it's usually nothing but empty carbs. Then, in an effort to be "good," they don't snack and maybe even eat a bare-bones salad at lunch. But all that noneating doesn't help them lose weight; in fact, it has the opposite effect because it *slows their metabolism down.* But now it's dinnertime and they're ravenous, so they're likely to consume far too many calories just as their metabolism has switched to its lowest gear. They overeat calories when their metabolism is at its weakest.

WHAT *IS* YOUR METABOLISM?

Now that I've thrown it around a few times, it's worth taking a minute to talk about what the word *metabolism* means. I think it may be one of the most abused words in the dieting industry. Lots of "experts" use it in a smoke-and-mirrors way that makes weight loss sound far more complicated than it is.

Our metabolism—the way we convert chemicals in our body into energy—is, *to some degree,* something we're stuck with, thanks to genetics. But we can—and must, if we want to lose weight—raise our metabolic rate. Two proven ways to boost it are exercise (especially weight-bearing exercise, which we'll talk more about in Chapter 8) and eating smaller, more frequent meals—in other words, snacking!

And what is the best way to slow our metabolism down, so

that it conserves energy and burns fewer calories, and so that it holds on to the weight we want to lose in our stomach and tush? Eating too little or eating too infrequently. Missing a single meal is enough to signal to our bodies that we might be on the verge of a famine, and our metabolism slows to compensate.

People spend a lot of time complaining about this trait, but it's actually a good thing—or at least it was 10,000 years or so ago. Genetic researchers believe that human beings developed this tendency—which they call the "thrifty gene"— back when we were hunters and gatherers. (Actually, our eating is influenced by about two hundred genes, which work together to control eating behavior and weight regulation, though probably only five to fifteen genes play key roles, researchers say. These genes control the production of important digestive hormones like ghrelin, which tells us when we're hungry, and leptin, which signals when we're full.) So hours-long stretches without eating tilt us into "thrifty" mode, anticipating a drastic cut in our daily ration of nuts, roots, and whatever else the cave people may have noshed on.

In some genetic groups, such as the Pima Indians in the Southwest, this ability to store fat efficiently is quite pronounced. While it probably worked well when food was gathered traditionally, it's not the best evolutionary adaptation in modern times when high-calorie foods are available around the clock, 365 days a year. It has caused terrible health problems for the Pima: roughly 50 percent of them are diabetic, and in 95 percent of those cases, they are also overweight.

While they are an extreme example, the lesson applies to all of us. We're genetically programmed to live in a feast-or-famine world, but are lucky enough to live in a country with the safest, most affordable and abundant food supply in the history of man. That's great news for keeping the nation chugging along, but not so great for those of us who don't need to store fat in our butts in case of famine. Snacking is the solution.

HUNGER VERSUS APPETITE

Part of the problem is that so many of us confuse hunger with appetite, when they're really very different. Nutrition researchers have found that there are three main components to appetite that control how much, how often, and the kinds of food we eat:

1. Hunger—when our body is truly saying, "Feed me *now*— I'm running on empty!"

2. Fullness—literally, how full our stomachs feel, which is why foods like popcorn (high in fiber) and chicken (high in protein) leave us with a different sense of satiety than pretzels or bagels (which are nonnutrient dense).

3. Desire to eat—this one confuses people, who sometimes think, "But it tastes so good to me. It must mean I'm hungry for it." This is very dangerous territory. If crème brûlée is your thing, for instance, it will taste good to you 24/7, whether you're truly hungry or not. (Of course, there are times when you just want to eat—we'll discuss that in Chapter 6, and I promise you'll get your indulgences!)

GETTING IN TOUCH WITH YOUR INNER HUNGER

My advice to clients who are having a hard time getting back in touch with their HQ is to think like a kid again. For parents, this is easy. If you don't have kids, spend a little time watching someone else's four-year-old, and you'll notice a wonderful pattern. Most kids *only* eat when they're hungry. (Of course, that doesn't include the kids who have been allowed to eat junk all day!) Stick a plate of pasta in front of a child who's not ready to eat yet—even if it's his favorite food in the whole wide world—and he may build a mountain, make tunnels, or feed it to the dog. But he won't eat a bite.

Even when they are hungry, kids eat differently than adults. Most won't take an extra serving of potatoes just because the bowl is on the table. On some days, they may push their broccoli away; other days, they may eat twice as much as usual.

It works the other way, too. If the parents' errand schedule has deprived a child of food for too long, everyone within earshot knows it. Hungry children quickly get crabby (and younger ones may even pitch world-class tantrums) until Mom or Dad wises up and produces the requisite bag full of Cheerios. The same thing happens to hungry adults—we just don't admit it. We blame our bad moods on delayed flights or long lines instead of realizing that the only thing wrong with our day is that we haven't eaten enough.

But we need to reconnect with those hunger cues because it's how those naturally thin people stay that way—like children, they listen to their bodies. Have you ever wondered about those lucky people who can, and often do, order a slice of pizza and then stop at just one slice? They don't act out some drama dance inside their head—"I should have pizza; no, I shouldn't have pizza!" "I had a slice—may as well just devour the whole pie!" These naturally thin people know how to keep food choices simple. They say, "I *love* pizza! And that hit the spot—it was just what I needed." Yes, I promise you, people like that *do* exist, and you can be one of them.

It just means being open-minded enough to rethink the timing of your meals. Later in the book we will talk about backing away from black-and-white eating ("I had a bag of M&Ms, so I might as well have ice cream, too; the whole day is shot anyway"). First, I'd like you to think about black-and-white timing. Suppose you're at work, and all around you people are sending out for skimpy salads, but you feel hungry enough for a bigger meal—maybe even a "dinner" type of meal, such as a pork chop. Have it! A piece of protein (with fat trimmed, don't forget . . .) with vegetables is likely to pack on fewer calories than a salad loaded with high-calorie toppings! Later in the day, when you used to grab something from the vending machine, listen to your body: it's not just craving calories. Those hunger pangs are a cry for help, not Swedish Fish! Eat a yogurt and a small handful of nuts, and see how much better you feel. And when it's dinnertime, your spouse may want to sit down to an 800-calorie meal. But chances are, you'll be more than happy with a chicken breast, a salad, and steamed vegetables. In fact, this is the way Europeans have been eating for centuries, and it's one of the main reasons they are so much less likely to be overweight than Americans.

If you are like many of my clients, this is the point when you fold your arms across your chest and shake your head. "As if," you're thinking. "I cannot imagine how a meal that includes salad *and* steamed vegetables will ever make me happy."

"Maybe," I'll say. But then I ask them to make just one change in their behavior in the week ahead: on a scale of 1 to 10, 1 being "stuffed" and 10 being "famished," I ask them to try to keep their HQ between a 4 and a 6 at all times. I tell them I don't even care what they eat; I just want them to become aware of their fluctuating HQ.

WHAT'S YOUR HQ?

1. Stuffed (to the point   *I'm never eating again!*
   of not feeling well)

2. Extremely full   *I couldn't eat another bite!*

3. Satisfied   *Could have skipped those last few bites!*

4. Slightly satisfied   *I feel satisfied with not one bit of fullness.*

5. Neutral   *I'm not hungry or full.*

6. Slightly hungry   *I guess I am about ready to eat, or I could have a few more bites.*

7. Hungry   *I'm really ready for another meal.*

8. Very hungry   *I'm definitely ready for a big meal!*

9. Extremely hungry   *I can't do one more thing until I eat!*

10. Famished (ready to pass out)   *Don't talk to me until I eat— I could eat my shirt!*

FACTOR THIS!

WHAT'S ALL THIS I KEEP HEARING ABOUT LEPTIN?

Leptin is a hormone manufactured in fat cells. It sends a signal to the brain that we've received enough nourishment and that it's time to stop eating. When it was first discovered about a decade ago, researchers thought it might be a huge breakthrough in treating obesity. But after millions of dollars in development, efforts to use leptin as a diet drug have been a major disappointment. In fact, it turns out that overweight people may already have more leptin, but that somehow, the "time to stop eating" message just doesn't make it to the brain as effectively as it does in thinner people. Experts still think drugs with leptin may turn out to help dieters—eventually. Recently, researchers at the University of Pittsburgh learned that C-reactive protein, an indicator of inflammation in the body that is elevated in overweight people, binds to leptin and interferes with its ability to control our eating. Stay tuned!

WHAT'S YOUR BODY *REALLY* SAYING?

Within a day or so, my clients report that it's easier to come up with an accurate HQ number, and they realize they've been misreading many of their body's hunger signals. It can take a while to figure out. Lots of times, they'll see that they aren't hungry at all, but are really thirsty. A glass of water—with a squirt of fresh lemon juice for flavor—is often all your body really needs.

More often, they're bored. Most of us rely on our eating habits to break up the monotony of a long day or a boring task at work. Sometimes, what seems like hunger is just our body's way of asking for a break from nonstop stress. I've had clients tell me that a quick walk around the block is what they really needed, just long enough to grab some fresh air and a little reprieve from the daily office drama.

The HQ scale also helps people get in touch with whether or not they're engaging in emotional eating. Researchers have been studying this behavior—in people who eat to help them manage feelings of anger, frustration, anxiety, or depression—for years in conjunction with eating disorders. But you don't need to have an eating disorder to eat this way. In fact, it's probably been a coping mechanism since childhood, and in its mildest form, there's nothing wrong with it—if the occasional ice cream cone helps a normal-weight person shake off the blues, what's the harm? But for people who routinely use food as a way to deal with their feelings, it's a strategy that quickly turns into unwanted pounds as the "occasional" ice cream cone evolves into an everyday routine. Studies have shown that people in this category—particularly women, for reasons researchers don't yet fully understand—also eat differently when they're under more stress.

FACTOR THIS!

I DON'T FEEL LIKE EATING ALL DAY. BUT THEN ALL OF A SUDDEN, I'M HUNGRY ENOUGH TO EAT A SMALL CHILD!

I bet you've been avoiding your body's phone calls. Even if you don't feel hungry, take a break midmorning and midafternoon: get up, stretch, have a drink of water. Ask yourself, "Am I hungry?" Try something light and small just to get your metabolism going. I think you'll see you do feel hungry and need to eat.

PUTTING YOUR HQ TO THE TEST

Here's an example from one of my client's first food journals. Susan came to me because she had been struggling to lose fifteen pounds for the last several years. Check out her HQ scores and the relationship between her level of hunger and the quality of her food choices.

Client: Susan   **Age:** 33   **Height:** 5'5"   **Weight:** 145 lbs.
Profession: Attorney

BREAKFAST: 8:30 A.M. at desk
    HQ 7   Mood: Good
½ cinnamon-raisin bagel, 1 tablespoon cream cheese, coffee and skim milk

LUNCH: 3:30 P.M. (she got stuck in court!) walking back to office
    HQ 9   Mood: Tense
2 slices of pizza, Diet Coke

DINNER: 8:30 P.M. at home (worked all afternoon; ran a few errands after work)
    HQ 8   Mood: Exhausted

Leftover chicken chow mein, ½ pint Ben & Jerry's Cherry Garcia Low-fat Frozen Yogurt, Water

You may think she sounds a little extreme, but many of my clients, whether attorneys like Susan, creative types who make their own schedules, or stay-at-home moms, are this busy. They have to work in meals around demanding schedules, and like Susan, they have very little time to make smart food decisions. And I'm not just talking about calories or fat (although this particular day gave Susan way too much of both, and not nearly enough of the fiber-rich carbohydrates, lean proteins, healthy fats, or nourishing antioxidant-high vegetables she needs). I'm more worried about Susan's blood sugar level. If I were to plot it, it would look like a roller coaster!

Erratic blood sugar levels affect many aspects of health, but especially mood. Who would have thought that a day that included pizza, Chinese food, *and* ice cream could have resulted in her feeling grouchy for hours? This roller-coaster ride also left her feeling wiped out when she needed the energy the most: in court, and then back at her office. It contributed to her feeling so exhausted that when she got home, instead of getting together with friends or reading a good book, or perhaps going to the gym, she ate her dinner standing over the kitchen counter and then collapsed on the couch with TiVo.

Because Susan has consumed her calories in an irregular pattern, Mother Nature has played a mean trick: even though Susan spent most of the day feeling hungry, her body burned far fewer calories than it should have, completely undermining her weight-loss goals. (Remember, this is a woman who started her day virtuously, with *half* a bagel.) Registered Dieticians (R.D.s) like me have suspected this for a long time, but researchers in the U.K. recently proved it. A group of healthy-weight women were given the same number of calories per day, but some were told to consume them in six intervals (similar to the Snack Factor Diet), some in three intervals, and some in nine. After a week of each, subjects were then told to fast overnight, so researchers could measure their true resting metabolic rate (or how fast their body was burning calories). Women who ate more sporadically—like Susan, consuming more calories in fewer sittings, and at unpredictable times—had a significant reduction in "thermic effect." Translation: the calories just sat there, waiting to be converted to a larger jean size, instead of getting burned up as energy, as they should have. (The same researchers have found similar results with overweight women as well.)

With all that in mind, at our next appointment, we improved Susan's breakfast to include more fiber and protein. Then we made sure she carried snacks in her bag at all times, so that she could have something on the way to or from court, if necessary. And at work, because it often happens that she can't take even ten minutes to run out for a bite, she now keeps almonds at her desk in individual snack-size Ziplocs and stocks the fridge there with drinkable yogurts.

A sample day from Susan's second week:

BREAKFAST: 8:30 A.M. at desk
    HQ 7   Mood: Good
1 slice whole wheat toast, 1 hard-boiled egg, 1 Starbucks Tall Skim Latte

SNACK: 10:30 A.M. (on the way to court)
    HQ 6   Mood: Good
10 almonds, a drinkable yogurt

LUNCH: 3:30 P.M.
    HQ 7   Mood: A little hassled

Mixed green salad, Grilled chicken, 1 tablespoon Italian dressing, 1 small apple, water

SNACK: 5:00 P.M.
    HQ 5   Mood: Good
KeriBar (I started manufacturing these bars because I wanted my clients to have an all-natural snack that provides protein, fiber, and healthy fats for maximum satiety, and I donate a percentage of the proceeds to fight childhood obesity.)
Herbal tea

DINNER: 8:30 P.M. at home
    HQ 8   Mood: Relaxed
Grilled chicken sausage, mixed green salad with 1 tablespoon vinaigrette, steamed broccoli, 1 cup blueberries, water

See how something as simple as paying attention to her HQ and snacking started a domino effect of healthy changes? Susan had the energy to fuel herself in court. And she is burning calories. It also allowed her to make a healthy decision on her way back to the office. Instead of feeling as if she were on the verge of stealing the sausage pizza from the corner pizzeria, she was able to walk right past it to the deli and pick out something else that appealed to her. And the KeriBar she ate while she was cleaning up some paperwork at the office gave her enough healthy energy for her to make it to the supermarket and pick up the sausage she'd been craving (albeit in a healthier chicken form), as well as enough other healthy food to stock her kitchen to get her through the rest of the week. Even though this wasn't a *perfect* Snack Factor day, just by adding two little snacks, Susan made a dramatic improvement in her diet and set herself up to succeed at every level. It's no surprise to me that she dropped three pounds in her first week of snacking well alone.

And even though she ate more often, she ate less overall. And Susan is typical: in one study, obesity researchers found that after just two weeks of adding a 210-calorie snack before an evening meal, participants were likely to eat an average of 300 calories less in the next meal. And the snackers felt more satiated after these smaller meals as well. This is why I always say that *snacks anchor your health*—and your weight—keeping it on an even keel and making dieting smooth sailing.

In the following weeks on the Snack Factor Diet, Susan made progressively healthier food choices, allowing her to keep her hunger and blood sugar levels stable and to lose weight at a healthy pace. She's down to her goal weight of 130, and she has figured out a way to plan her meals so that she has a slice of pizza for lunch each week.

Here's a look at a sample day from another client, Robert, now in his fourth week of the Snack Factor Diet. Unlike Susan, whose work schedule could get pretty zany, Robert sits behind a desk and has a predictable routine.

FACTOR THIS!

WHEN I EAT BREAKFAST, I AM HUNGRIER FOR LUNCH—SO I LIKE TO SKIP BREAKFAST.

When you eat breakfast, you're better prepared for the morning ahead. And the reason you're hungrier for lunch is that your *metabolism is working*! The reason you don't feel hungry for lunch when you skip breakfast is that you're deprived body is going into starvation mode—so you're not craving calories, but you're not burning any, either. So eat breakfast and have a midmorning snack to help keep you on track when lunchtime comes.

Name: Robert   **Age:** 37   **Height:** 6'0"   **Weight:** 225
Profession: Investment Banker

BREAKFAST: 7:00 A.M.

   HQ 8   Mood: Good
1 slice whole wheat toast, 4-egg-white omelet, Starbucks Grande Skim Latte

LUNCH: 11:45 A.M.

   HQ 6   Mood: Good (out at business lunch—he does this
   3–4 times per week)
Mixed green salad with onions, tomatoes, carrots, 1 tablespoon vinaigrette dressing; 8-ounce grilled tuna; steamed green beans; seltzer with lime

SNACK: 2:00 P.M.

   HQ 6   Mood: Somewhat stressed
Dannon Light & Fit Yogurt (they sell them in his office building), 10 almonds, water

SNACK: 4:00 P.M.

   HQ 5   Mood: Anxious to finish up something for work
Celery sticks and 2 teaspoons peanut butter

DINNER: 7:30 P.M.

   HQ 4   Mood: Great
8-ounce steak filet, tomato and onion salad with 1 ounce blue cheese and balsamic vinegar, large bowl steamed spinach, large seltzer, 1 light beer

What's exciting to me about Robert's daily routine now isn't just that it's allowed him to knock off eleven pounds—it's that he's feeling great doing it. Because he's done some experimenting and found the right timing for him; by the end of the day his HQ is at a very comfortable 4, and his metabolism has been steadily stoked.

HOW SNACKING CHANGES BEHAVIOR

Much of what I've mentioned so far deals with the physical science of snacking and weight loss—what's actually happening in your body when you choose almonds and yogurt over a bag of Lay's Baked potato chips. But what's as important (if not more so) is that snacking causes major behavioral changes, too. And after all, your behavior is the only thing that stands between you and the body weight you've been struggling to reach.

There's plenty of good science behind these behavioral claims. And I've seen it played out in my practice again and again. People who snack make better choices when they are

- **At restaurants.** Walking in with an HQ of 6, for example, allows you to be a cool customer, not someone waiting to wolf down the whole bread basket. You can sip a glass of water instead of obsessing about dinner rolls. And once those overly generous restaurant portions arrive, it's easier to remind yourself that there is no need to clean your plate—in fact, my clients quickly learn to eat about half of what they are served in most restaurants. You'll see those restaurant red-flag words like *fried, flaky,* or *puffed* for the fat traps they are and go for something grilled instead. Or you'll make a conscious decision to have the house special you've been craving, but say no to dessert.

- **At parties.** With a day's worth of healthy snacks under their belts, my clients say they arrive and survey the food that's laid out as someone who's ready to pick and choose

among the best of the spread, not a desperado monopoliz-
ing the chips and dips.

- **In grocery stores.** Don't go in hungry—have a snack before you start shopping. Try not to shop at a time of day
when you're emotional or hungry; if you're always tired
and grouchy at the end of a workday, save shopping for
Saturday mornings. You are more likely to buy junk and
things you don't need when you shop at these times. And
most people get themselves in trouble when they start
browsing. I suggest you have two lists, one with bare essen-
tials for a quick trip and one that's more elaborate for
when you have the time.

- **At home.** People who come home starved at the end of the
day are vulnerable. They often wind up inhaling the first
thing they get their hands on—sometimes even food they
don't really like—because the idea of chopping even a
single vegetable makes them want to lie down and pass
out. (Remember that four-year-old we talked about? It's
no surprise that so many tantrums happen just before
dinner!) But when you've been giving your body what it
needs, right when it needs it, dinner isn't that overwhelm-
ing. Even after a rough day, you can summon the strength
to defrost a piece of chicken, steam some frozen vegetables,
and eat at the table like a human being, instead of gulping
down three-day-old leftovers in front of the fridge. Healthy
"clean" meals are more appealing when you have not deprived yourself all day.

- **At the table.** Snacking allows you to eat more slowly and
therefore consume less food. That's because it takes about
twenty minutes for leptin and other digestive chemicals to
kick in and send signals to the brain that say, "Whoa—I've

had enough." If you've always been a speed-eater, it's not a habit you'll change overnight. It's going to take some conscious effort on your part. My clients tell me it helps them to put their fork down in between bites, for example, or sip water often throughout the meal.

If you're *starving*, with an HQ of 7 or more, this kind of slow, deliberate eating is torture. But if you've snacked well, it's rewarding. In fact, some people find this style of eating not just healthful but also spiritual. Mindful eating is a practice that's gaining favor among meditation teachers around the country, and is even taught at trendy spas like Miraval in Tucson, Arizona. The idea—like all mindfulness practices—is to breathe deeply, taste your food fully, and really savor it. When you're thinking about nothing else but the food in your mouth, you're living fully in the moment. For those who practice regularly, those kinds of mindfulness meditations are proven stress reducers, which not only help you manage your weight, but also boost your immune system. And if that all sounds a little too New Agey, fine. But mindful eating will definitely put you in closer touch with your HQ and closer to that strapless dress you can't wait to wear again!

2

Thinking in Thirds:

Keeping Everything in Proportion

The "right" proportion of foods (the ratios of carbohydrate to fat to protein) shifts as often and dramatically as hemlines in this country. Over three decades ago, cardiologist Dr. Robert Atkins published *Dr. Atkins' Diet Revolution* (yes—he first hit the scene in 1972, a year when both miniskirts and maxiskirts were in vogue!) and was one of the early proponents of a high-protein diet. But as doctors began to worry about all the animal fat and cholesterol Americans were consuming, nutrition experts began urging people to limit protein (because most people were focusing on animal proteins, which are high in saturated fat) and to eat more and more carbohydrate. Fat was believed to be the enemy of the national waistline, not calories.

But unlike the Atkins diet (or the Scarsdale, or the grapefruit, or any number of popular diets at that time), the low-fat, high-carb approach to eating was no fad. In fact, it was practically law, cemented in 1992 by no less an authority than the

U.S. Department of Agriculture (USDA). (The USDA has been in charge of setting nutritional guidelines for America since the 1890s.) America went nuts for anything with "low-fat" or "nonfat" slapped on the label.

It's not that low-fat or nonfat foods are bad—foods that are naturally low in fat are among the healthiest. It's just that Americans were all too willing to embrace a "low-fat food" even if it was also low in nutrition and high in calories. For example, I remember in college, the low-fat frenzy fueled a bin-candy craze, when I developed a real fondness for Sour Patch Kids and Swedish Fish. Candies that were more or less 100 percent sugar sounded almost like health food with those "fat-free food" stickers on the bags! And who could forget the Snackwell's cookie obsession? After Nabisco introduced them in 1994, supermarkets had to struggle to keep the devil's food cookies—just as high in calories as other cookies—on the shelves, and even took out national ads to apologize for the shortage!

There was just one problem: the more Americans followed this all-carbs-are-good-carbs, all-fat-is-bad-fat style of eating, the heavier people got. Between 1991, just before the USDA introduced the Food Pyramid, and 2000, America's low-fat eating helped fuel a colossal weight gain. The number of overweight adults in America increased 61 percent, according to the Centers for Disease Control.

Worse, by not paying attention to the little fat they did eat, they missed out on important nutrition. Fat is essential to a healthy diet, not just because it transports fat-soluble vitamins, and provides cushioning and insulation, but also because our body requires fat for our metabolism to function properly. Studies have shown that when people eat too little fat, it actually slows down their weight-loss efforts. In short, we need fat to burn fat. Researchers have found that some fats, including many of the types I recommend here, can actually boost your metabolism because the body uses them more readily as energy than other fats.

It wasn't long before the pendulum started swinging the other way. Dieters who tried hard to follow the guidelines dictated in the Food Pyramid found it tough—sometimes impossible—to lose weight. Not surprisingly, when the Atkins diet was republished in 1992, it took only a few years before it had again become the center of the national weight-loss debate. Through Atkins' radically different diet from the USDA's—and one that many doctors warned was downright dangerous—some Americans began to lose weight. And as more and more of these "dangerous" dieters succeeded, the conventional experts had to concede the point: by eating as the USDA recommended, the typical American was gaining weight.

Adding to the confusion was the way people began tossing diet descriptions around. Lots of people, for example, called Atkins-style diets "low-carb," which is accurate, but also "high-protein," which was misleading. In reality, a typical Atkins-type day provided a moderate amount of protein (about 33 percent). The real imbalance was the scarcity of carbs (about 3 percent of daily calories) and the abundance of fats (about 64 percent of daily calories).

Whatever you called it, this low-carb craze wasn't much of a solution, either. While plenty of people lost a considerable amount of weight on diets like Atkins or Sugar Busters, it usually came galloping back as soon as the dieters went back to their normal routines. That's what happens with any overly restrictive meal plan: you're counting the days until you can go back to "normal," when normal was what got you overweight in the first place! (Researchers call this the "restraint theory," and have found that people who diet in this restrictive way are more likely to go on occasional food binges than those who don't.) And increasingly, the evidence began showing that the Atkins diet potentially created serious health risks.

This rebounding was especially true with many Atkins adherents' drastic reduction in all carbs—good carbs such as whole grains as well as nonnutrient-dense carbs. Many people convinced themselves that the type of fats they ate, whether the pork rinds, sour cream, and bacon allowed by Atkins or the heart-healthy oils like olive oil and canola oil proposed by the more health-conscious experts, were one and the same.

By 2005, America's obsession with the low-carb craze had pretty much run its course—Atkins' company even filed for bankruptcy. Our infatuation with low-fat diets was clearly pretty much kaput, too. The Women's Health Initiative released a massive study that showed that low-fat diets didn't provide many of the health benefits people expected, either. Women eating a lower-fat diet were just as likely to get breast cancer, colorectal cancer, and even heart disease as women who didn't eat the lower-fat diet. That same year, the USDA issued new guidelines to replace the Food Pyramid. In many ways, these are a huge improvement. They spell out quite clearly which fats are better than others, and they encourage the consumption of whole grains over simple, sugary carbs.

But still the guidelines continue to be confusing because carbs, protein, and fats appear in so many foods. Experts like me worry that these guidelines are still not helpful to people looking for weight-loss guidance. In fact, that's why I use the word *starch* to make it clear that foods like bread, legumes, and cereal are in a different category from other carbohydrate-rich foods like fruit or your evening glass of chardonnay.

The percentages are still maddeningly vague, and you al-

most have to be a private eye to find out what the current recommendations are. If you were to sit down right now and
Google your way through every government Web site you could
find (how much like fun does that sound?), it might take
you decades to discover that the new USDA guidelines recommend that only about 18 percent of calories per day come
from protein sources. That's in spite of increasing evidence
that a moderate consumption of protein promotes weight loss
as well as weight maintenance.

And it's just downright confusing that the Institute of
Medicine, another government-funded organization of scientists that tracks nutrients and health, says that eating anywhere from 10 to 35 percent protein is healthy. Who could
blame people for throwing up their hands and saying, "I don't
know who to believe anymore!"

That's why so many people have diets that are so radically
off the mark. Some people, struggling to lose weight, wander
through each day without a food compass. "I am a fat-free
junkie," a potential client will confess to me over the phone.
Or "I'm an Atkins addict . . . a binge eater . . . I'm Zoned
out." They've lost all perspective, and a typical day might include a breakfast muffin as big as Rhode Island ("But it's fat-
free," they say) or a dinner steak sized just right for Fred
Flintstone ("Hey, it was allowed on Atkins!"). But most often
they just say, "I want to be healthy. I'm sick and tired of being
so up and down and emotional about which eating plan I'm
on—or not on. I just want to feel good about what I am eating
and, of course, lose weight!"

And just as their "good" food list is off-kilter, so is their
"bad" food list. Sometimes, it takes real work for me to per-
suade my clients—at first—that, yes, their body needs fat,
and often it's more fat than they've been consuming. And
that while grapefruit does contain carbs (and sugar), it's also

loaded with fiber, vitamins, and phytonutrients. It's not fair to lump a grapefruit and a Pop-Tart in the same food group!

Let's end all the confusion, now. I recommend that people eat roughly a third of their daily calories in lean protein, another third in the best kinds of carbs, and the final third in heart-friendly fats. (Usually, they wind up eating a slightly higher percentage of carbs, which is perfectly natural and absolutely fine.) It's a sensible, moderate guideline that has allowed hundreds of my clients to lose weight.

A HEALTHY BALANCE: THINKING IN THIRDS

It is time to get "proportioned!" As soon as I sit down with a new client, I teach the person that he or she should never write off entire food groups, but instead pick and choose among all of them for the foods that provide the most nutrition, satisfaction, and pleasure. And I break down nutrition into three easy pieces to keep it simple. Over the course of a day, the client will be eating roughly equal proportions of carbs, proteins, and fats. Most days, he or she will be eating slightly more carbs from many food sources—we are not talking bread and pasta! Best of all, the day will be anchored by snacks that provide just what he or she is craving, just when they are needed the most.

There are two reasons I promote this formula of roughly one third/one third/one third (remember: slightly more carbs):

1. *It's simple.* No matter how hard other diet experts try to make it, it is easier than you think. There is no calorie counting, no math to be done, no index cards to arrange, no measuring and weighing, and no points to add up! This is a lifestyle—something you should be able to follow whether you are at home in restaurant-rich New York City, on the

range in Wyoming, in organic northern California, or anywhere else in our "fast-food nation."

2. *It works.* After decades of research, the bulk of evidence now points to an eating path that is halfway between the no-fat and low-carb pendulum swings that America's been caught up in. Moderate-protein diets, with a reasonable amount of good carbohydrates and the appropriate amount of healthy fat, are the best way to lose weight and the most effective way to maintain weight loss. For one thing, thanks to the Institute of Medicine, we know that eating a third of the day's calories from protein is safe. For another, more and more studies have found that increasing protein consumption—to moderate levels, of course—is more likely to result in weight-loss success.

Here's some of the latest evidence that diets providing a moderate amount of protein (33 percent or so, as I recommend here) are healthy, safe, and effective:

• Researchers at the University of Washington in Seattle recently took a group of healthy people and put half of them on a lower-protein (15 percent of daily calories) regimen and the other half on a higher-protein diet (30 percent of daily calories). For the first two weeks, the diets were controlled, and those on the higher-protein plan lost more weight and reported feeling higher levels of satiety than those stuck on the lower-protein plan. But the best part was that, in the experiment's final two weeks, participants were told they could eat as much as they wanted as long as they honored the protein percentage they were assigned. The 30 percent-protein group continued to feel significantly more satiety, and as a result consumed an average of 441 calories fewer per day. So they continued to lose weight even though they were no longer "on a diet."

- Swapping protein for carbohydrates has been shown to improve blood lipids. One Harvard University study looked at more than 900 cases of heart disease in women over a fourteen-year period, whose protein intake ranged from 14 percent of daily calories to 24 percent. Researchers found that a lower-protein diet actually *increased* the risk of heart disease.

- An analysis from a group of researchers in the Netherlands determined that moderate-protein diets are more effective for weight loss. The number one reason, the authors found, comes back to that one little buzzword I introduced back in the Introduction: *satiety*. Second, they learned that more protein consumption makes us more likely to burn calories from fat (and isn't that what we all want—to burn the excess from our thighs?).

- These same researchers also found that eating more protein makes it easier to keep the weight off. Dieters who increased their protein intake to 18 percent of daily calories from 15 percent regained only half as much weight as those eating just 15 percent in protein.

- At the Harvard School of Public Health, researchers recently sifted through more than fifty previously published studies, and found that this moderate-protein type of eating "exerts an increased thermic effect." The more protein we eat, the more calories we burn. And these diets are definitely more effective for weight loss over a six-month period. (The jury is still out on longer-term results, but many more studies are now underway.)

Eating in thirds makes sense to my clients. And because I am not asking them to severely limit their fat intake, I know they will find it much easier to stay with the Snack Factor Diet while enjoying plenty of delicious foods. My proudest moments usually happen about thirty days into the diet, when clients tell me the best news any nutritionist can hear. "This doesn't even feel like a diet anymore," they'll say. "This is just how I live now. This is just the way I want to eat."

That's because the third/third/third formula is a natural way to eat, and that ratio occurs in so many satisfying food combinations. Plenty of foods you already love—not foods you'll have to force yourself to tolerate—break down in just this proportion. Most people find this balance satisfying in terms of providing that quick burst of energy and satisfying hunger for several hours. So there's no math; it's a matter of eating the way you naturally like to eat. The roughly equal thirds will just happen after a little more guidance.

Of course, lots of good snacks, especially those that people grab on the go, may be less balanced. A hard-boiled egg or a handful of almonds provides protein and fat, but no real carbs; a low-sugar nonfat drinkable yogurt will offer protein and carbs, but no fat. That's just fine. Not every morsel of food you eat has to fit this pattern—but if you follow the Snack Factor Diet, at the end of the day you will hit these proportions.

Don't believe me? Here's a typical Snack Factor day:

BREAKFAST
½ cup Kellogg's All-Bran Extra Fiber
1 tablespoon chopped walnuts
1 cup skim milk

SNACK
2 celery sticks
2 teaspoons Arrowhead Mills natural peanut butter

LUNCH
Spinach salad with broccoli, celery, and cucumbers
4 ounces steamed shrimp

¼ avocado
Dijon vinaigrette dressing

SNACK
1 FAGE Total 0% Yogurt
12 almonds

DINNER
Chicken Parmesan (4 ounces grilled chicken, ½ cup
    Colavita Marinara Sauce, 3 tablespoons grated Parmesan
    cheese)
Steamed asparagus
Chopped salad with romaine lettuce, red onions, green
    peppers, carrots
Balsamic and lemon dressing

If you're the kind of person who just said, "Wait—that's
not equal thirds," we need to have a little chat. No, it's not
"perfect," and almost no day will be. (As I've said, overall,
for the next few weeks you'll probably find yourself eating
slightly more carbs.) But it's quite close. You need to trust
that as you learn to listen to your HQ and munch according to
plan, you'll naturally put yourself in the range of roughly
equal thirds—without a second thought. (Remember, I created this diet so people could relax and avoid stress about
what they are eating!)

ONE THIRD AT A TIME

Protein

The first building block is *protein*, which provides power
to the body in many ways. Not only is it the major structural
component of all cells of the body, but protein can function as
enzyme, hormone, and transporter/carrier. And while I've al-

ready explained why eating adequate amounts of lean protein will help you succeed at losing weight, here's how eating the Snack Factor way actually works.

At meals, protein-rich foods—as delicious as they are— seem to be easier for most of us to eat slowly, and then put on the brakes. Aim for lean proteins. Often, clients assume I make that recommendation for the most obvious reason: leaner proteins have less fat and therefore fewer calories, right? Absolutely. But there's an added bonus because lean proteins provide an extra boost to satiety levels. Swedish researchers found that when they gave a group of healthy-weight subjects a serving of fish (a lean protein) versus a serving of beef, the fish eaters felt somewhat more satiated. And as a result, at their next meal they ate, on average, 11 percent fewer calories than the beef eaters.

So experiment with some of these lean proteins: egg whites, shrimp, turkey or chicken without the skin, fresh fish, or even canned tuna. Be adventurous. Lean cuts of pork or beef are both good choices and will keep you from feeling as if your choices are too restrictive.

FACTOR THIS!

THE SKINNY ON TUNA

Chunk light is the best choice of tuna because it has the lowest level of mercury—in general, compared with white tuna, chunk light has one third as much mercury. But a recent study did find that 6 percent of the chunk light sampled contained the same level of mercury or higher than white. The FDA has not changed warnings because they believe that the levels do not pose a significant threat. However, many obstetricians caution pregnant women to avoid tuna altogether owing to uncertainty. Check out www.vitalchoice.com for excellent sources of low-mercury tuna.

Carbohydrates

Carbohydrates, which include sugars (such as those found in fruit) and starches (like those found in bread, cereal, and vegetables like corn, potatoes, and beans), provide energy to the cells of the body, particularly the brain. While protein and fat provide the body with backup stores of energy, carbohydrates are what we turn into fuel first. That's why we get that burst of energy shortly after eating a carb-rich food, and so many of us crave it when we feel lethargic!

But again, all carbs are not equal, which is why the energy burst we get from a 100-calorie banana (that's one of those really *big* bananas; smaller ones have about 60 calories) feels so much more pleasant than the manic jolt we get from one of those nutrient-deficient 100-calorie cookie packs.

The Snack Factor Diet focuses on high-fiber carbohydrates. Most of the carbs I suggest will be delicious whole grains: hot and cold cereals for breakfast, fiber-rich crackers, or even protein-rich carbs, such as chickpeas or black or red beans. After the first four weeks, you'll also have one serving of fruit per day, whether you choose a pear in the morning or a cup of berries with cottage cheese for an afternoon snack.

I'll be honest. For the first few days you may miss some of your old carb friends—the big bagels, the bottomless pots of pasta, the garlic bread the waiter never stops bringing. And if you're someone with a strong sweet tooth, you may miss those simple sugars as well. But as your HQ gets stronger, you'll feel those pangs less and get smarter about satisfying them.

To an extent, we can "trick" that sweet tooth. There's no shortage of products with artificial sweeteners, from diet sodas to cookies to breakfast cereals and ice creams. I warn people to avoid them as much as possible. In the beginning, I tell my clients it's okay to occasionally have a diet soda, especially if it gets you through a tough time at a restaurant. Or if you struggle to consume enough water, it's OK (but *not* recommended) to use products like Crystal Light to get in your fluids. But I'd rather have you drink water and lemon or seltzer with lime. It's important to be careful because the real problem is that many of us have become too attached to sickly sweet foods. So while a diet soda is a fine crutch once in a while, it's not doing anything to help your body recover its taste for naturally sweet foods. On the Snack Factor Diet I want you to feel healthy, clean, and natural as you lose weight. Within a week or so, a glass of plain water with natural flavors (for example, just a packet of True Lemon) will taste like the most refreshing beverage in the world to you.

FACTOR THIS!

WHAT'S THE DEAL WITH DIET SODA AND ARTIFICIAL SWEETENERS?

I urge people to do all they can to completely avoid artificial sweeteners. For example, I would rather you drink seltzer with lemon than a diet cola. I always tell my clients to imagine that they've just had a massage at a luxurious, exclusive spa. What are you thirsty for—a cool glass of lemon water with its pure, clean ingredients? Or a diet soda with its absolutely unpronounceable list of chemical additives? While diet sodas won't add any calories, they do expose your body to all kinds of chemicals you don't need. Even worse, these sweeteners just cause you to crave more sweets and distort your natural sense of taste. Once you've gone a few days without them, you'll be amazed at how wonderfully sweet a grape, a blueberry, or even a tomato will taste!

That said, I would rather you save your sugar grams for whole food; for example, go for a handful of fresh blueberries instead of fruited yogurt. So if plain yogurt just doesn't have enough flavor for you, then it's OK to add a tiny bit of sweetener (versus grabbing fruited yogurt). However, just because they provide zero calories, sweeteners are not a

(continues)

free-for-all; my "lesser evil" favorites are Splenda and SweetLeaf Stevia. I will note whenever I recommend a product in the book that contains Splenda. (Please note that Stevia is *not* approved by the FDA as a sugar substitute and is considered a dietary supplement because it is an herb.)

Flavorful fats

Fat is a major source of energy for the body and aids in vitamin absorption and tissue development. Many studies have shown that of the three groups (protein, carboyhydrate, and fat), fats have the lowest ability to satiate our hunger—something that surprises many of my clients. "You're kidding?" they'll say. "Then what makes Häagen-Dazs seem so incredibly rich and satisfying to me?"

There are two reasons. One is that fat does provide some level of satiety; it's just not as much as proteins tend to. More important, though, fat greatly increases what experts call *palatability*—a fancy way of describing how appealing a food feels in our mouths. And yes, ice cream—thanks to its high fat content—does feel enormously appealing when we taste it, as do many other high-fat foods. Whether it's savory (like steak or bacon) or sweet (cake or cookies), these are the foods we give the ultimate compliment: *rich.* But these are also the easiest foods to overeat, and it doesn't take too many forkfuls for many of us to get into dangerous territory.

All that mouth appeal makes it easy to overdo fats, which is why experts have linked the consumption of highly palatable foods (especially those with a high sugar *and* high fat content) with overeating. Something about all that mouth-yumminess overrides our inborn satiety measures, so that we can eat way past the point of fullness. (If the term "pigging out" offends you, experts have given this kind of eating a slightly more highbrow name—they call it "passive overconsumption"!)

The cruel joke, of course, is that the more people indulge in these highly palatable foods, the more likely they are to gain weight, which in turn causes physiological changes that make it harder for them to lose weight. British researchers have found that as the rate at which the stomach empties changes, so does its hormonal response to food. That means the satiety response—the commonsense voice that might say, "OK, three cupcakes are more than enough!"—is much slower to kick in. (If it makes you feel any better, humans aren't the only ones drawn by the siren call of these high-fat, high-sugar foods. Researchers have shown that when rats are given the chance to choose such foods over their regular rat chow, they will take it, too.)

So it's not surprising to me when clients seem nervous about taking in a third or so of their calories each day from fat. (Believe it or not, I've had clients come to me who are quite overweight, but eat next to no fat!) Besides the endless hype about the benefits of low-fat eating, which we've already discussed, chances are good that they've had their own personal debacles with high-fat foods and don't quite trust themselves. (In fact, even people who don't normally describe their eating as "bingeing" often admit to some serious overeating of high-fat foods.)

But fat is vital to our health. It helps our bodies to function properly, and without it we'd be lost. Fat deficiency, although rare in the United States, causes dry skin, brittle hair and nails, chronic constipation and other forms of gastrointestinal distress, menstrual abnormalities, fatigue, anemia, impaired wound healing, soreness of the joints, headaches, and even memory loss. Besides, fat is yummy. It lends substance and flavor to the carbs and proteins we eat, and makes every snack and meal a little more satisfying. The foods I suggest on this plan are rich in monounsaturated and polyunsaturated fats, which have been shown to reduce blood cholesterol concentration and help lower the risk of heart disease. What's more, Snack Factor foods provide ample amounts of the essential fatty acids known as omega-3s—fats we desperately need, since our bodies are not able to manufacture them.

MY FAVORITE FAT

Researchers know that people who live in countries where plenty of fatty fish—like salmon and mackerel, both high in omega-3s—is consumed have less heart disease. (The longer-chain omega-6 fats are commonly found in vegetable oils, which can lower levels of low-density lipoprotein cholesterol [LDLs], which helps prevent heart disease. But most Americans already consume too many omega-6 fats, and overconsumption has been linked to irregular heart beats, blood clots, and certain types of cancer.)

FACTOR THIS!

A recent study published in the *American Journal of Clinical Nutrition* showed that salads with "regular" salad dressing versus salads with fat-free dressing promoted greater absorption of some nutrients.

I can't say enough about omega-3s. I recommend that my clients eat many foods that contain them, including salmon, sardines, flaxseed, and walnuts. That's because people who eat more of these healthy fats reduce their risk of death from a heart attack or stroke by at least 50 percent. The American Heart Association recommends that we include omega-3s in our diets regularly. A word of caution, though: at Harvard Medical School, researchers have found that when people are already suffering from angina or congestive heart failure, omega-3s may increase the risk of cardiac death. If you've had heart disease, talk to your doctor before adding too much fatty fish to your diet.

Many of my clients worry about all the bad stuff that can come from eating these fish, including pollutants like mercury and PCBs. And I do highly recommend that you try to eat wild salmon, which contains fewer harmful chemicals than farmed salmon, and eat farmed fish only occasionally. But please, don't let safety concerns scare you away from fish altogether. In fact, for middle-aged men and older, as well as for postmenopausal women, the benefits of eating omega-3s outweigh the risk of consuming too much mercury.

They may not be on everybody's regular shopping list, but I'm a big fan of sardines. One of my favorite sources of omega-3s is Nordic brisling sardines, which are fished from the cold, clean northern fjords. (Omega-3s break down in heat, so the farther north the fish comes from, the higher the concentration of omega-3s.) Not only do they offer a concentrated source of omega-3s—5.01 grams in a 3.50-ounce serving—they don't pose the same mercury or PCB risk as do larger ocean fish.

You won't find many of the "bad" fats on the Snack Factor Diet. You'll have very few saturated fats, trans fats, and dietary cholesterol, which are usually found in meats, bakery items, and full-fat dairy products. These heighten the risk of heart disease in some people by boosting the level of harmful, low-density lipoprotein cholesterol in the bloodstream, even with only very small quantities in the diet.

Of course, knowing that "good" fats are better for your heart is great. But there's another reason to work hard at learning to appreciate the joys of olive oil over, let's say, heavy cream. Researchers in Australia recently gave subjects a very high-fat breakfast, where 43 percent of calories came from fat. In one group, the foods eaten were enriched with olive oil, one of the best types of monounsaturated fats. Others ate a break-fast enriched with cream. Those with the monounsaturated-fat breakfast had a significantly higher fat oxidation rate (fat burned faster) than those who ate the "bad-fat" breakfast, meaning more of those calories were burned off.

Now that I've sold you (I hope!) on the importance of snacking, on keeping a close eye on your hunger, and on balancing proportions of protein, carbs, and fat, it's time to talk about the fun stuff—food! In the next chapter, we'll start to discuss which foods do the best job of keeping you satisfied.

Secrets of the Nutrient Bargain Hunter

Nutrient Density

From creamy bites of avocado, to toasted almonds, to satisfying steaks—what these foods have in common is that they provide your body with meaningful calories, delivering specific food components your body needs most. The technical term for this is *nutrient density:* the amount of and availability of nutrients found in a single food.

Just think back to the last time you grabbed a handful of M&Ms at a party. You probably ate 150 calories worth—about thirty-seven of those little melt-in-your-mouth wonders. But those are 150 empty calories, two-thirds sugar and one-third fat (all of it the kind you should be avoiding) and no fiber. So after that last crunchy mouthful, you were left with no nutritional reward for your efforts: the M&Ms gave your mouth a little lift, but they did nothing for the rest of your body.

So if you're like most people, as soon as you swallowed that harmless little 150-calorie serving, you probably (1) wanted more and resisted but spent the rest of the evening consciously avoiding the room where the hostess put the M&Ms, (2) gave in and ate another five handfuls and another 500 calories, or (3) had an extrabig slice of birthday cake. Those thirty-seven miserable M&Ms may have given you an instant sugar lift, but within a half hour, you were on a downward slope and began craving more sugar to fix it. They may not melt in your hand, but they don't provide any satiety, either.

In contrast, have you ever consumed 150 calories from a small apple and a spoonful of natural peanut butter? If you have, you could probably say that you (1) felt completely satisfied, (2) felt more energetic, and (3) made pretty good choices at your next meal. This is because an apple and peanut butter provide you with fiber, good fat, and protein, not to mention all of the other vitamins and minerals your body can use. It's a snack that satisfies every aspect of your appetite: your hunger, how full you feel, and your desire to eat something delicious. And because it kept your metabolism cranking, that snack probably held your HQ steady, so that you wanted to eat a healthy dinner that night, too.

Here's another way to look at it. Because my practice is in Manhattan, many of my clients pride themselves on being world-class shoppers who know a good deal when they see one. So it helps when we talk about nutrient density as a shopping decision. If you could spend $50 on a poorly made sweater that you knew would disintegrate after one use, or $150 on a beautiful cashmere sweater that you know would last for years, which would you pick?

Of course, that's a no-brainer: you'd recognize the well-made sweater for the bargain that it is. Well, on the Snack Factor Diet, you're going to learn to be a nutrient bargain hunter. Don't worry; you won't really count calories. (Although if it helps you to understand my approach, know that most people consume 1,200 to 1,600 calories a day on the stricter Snack Factor Diet, depending on how much they weigh, and slightly more after the first month.) But personally, I find counting calories boring and a little depressing. It would be like clothes shopping just by price tag, without thinking about what color a sweater is, how it fits, or how good it makes you feel when you slip it on.

So, yes, you will be choosing foods that are somewhat lower in calories. But you'll also be basing your decisions on nutrient density, and you'll choose your snacks as if you're going on a pleasant shopping challenge: you have a set amount to spend each day, but you must get the most nutrition for your money.

A QUICK WORD ABOUT THE GLYCEMIC INDEX (GI)

If you've read other diet or nutrition books, you probably know that nutrient density is sometimes related to a number called the *glycemic index* (GI) or *glycemic load.* While those numbers are important to nutritionists, as well as to people with diabetes and prediabetes, I tell my clients not to pay too much attention unless their doctors have asked them to. It's also problematic that the GI of foods changes when eaten with other foods and is confusing, since the portions of foods used for determining the GI are not the usual portion sizes. Frankly, I find that for most people, it's too easy to get confused by all the nutritional lingo, and it takes their eyes off the ball: as long as you're watching the four core components of the Snack Factor Diet—HQ, proportions, nutrient density, and portions—you'll stay in a healthy range. In fact, most Snack Factor foods happen to have a low score on this index, which is another way of saying that the carbs I recommend usually have more fiber and less sugar.

Let's face it: if you're already consciously monitoring the

foods you eat, why worry about one more set of numbers or more confusing terminology? Unless watching your diet is your full-time job (and how much fun would that be?), it's not realistic to have to look up everything you eat on a chart. By the time you finish this chapter, you'll fully understand the foods that provide you with high satiety and nutritional value, and you'll be able to use them as building blocks for an every-day game plan that works for you, giving you maximum eating satisfaction, blood sugar stabilization, and enjoyment—all without having to think as if you've got a Ph.D. in food chemistry!

FILL UP ON FIBER!

One of the most important things to know about any food's nutrient density is how much fiber it has. Although fiber doesn't contain any nutrients (we actually can't even digest it!), it helps keep us healthy in several ways. While the science of fiber study is relatively new, early indications are that consuming adequate amounts of fiber may lower cholesterol and prevent certain cancers. Doctors are so bullish on fiber's ability to help control blood sugar levels that they recommend that people with diabetes eat even more fiber than the rest of us—up to 50 grams per day, compared to the overall recommendations of 20 to 35 grams (38 grams for men ages 14–50) for other adults. Fiber also prevents constipation, diverticulosis, and hemorrhoids.

Because fiber is found primarily in plant-based foods, consuming a higher-fiber diet also helps ensure that you're getting your fair share of vitamins, minerals, and phyto-chemicals (powerful compounds in plant-based foods that help keep our immune system strong). Good sources of fiber tend to be low in fat and rich in nutrients.

You've probably even heard people discuss types of fiber: *soluble* (that's the kind in oat bran, which is thought to help lower blood cholesterol levels and regulate the body's use of sugars) and *insoluble* (found in fruits and vegetables, which aid in digestion and prevent constipation by adding bulk and softness to stools). But the more nutritionists learn about the benefits of fiber, the less impressed they are with the benefits of one type over another, and the National Academy of Sciences has recommended that the two terms be phased out in favor of plain old *fiber.*

However you categorize it, the best news about fiber is that it fills you up, and you tend to feel more satisfied. Fiber-rich foods score higher on the satiety index than others. That's why a nutty whole-grain bread, for example, feels so much more satisfying after we've eaten it than white bread, or a juicy pear stays with us so much longer than a handful of pretzels.

If you want the nitty-gritty details, scientists believe that there are several reasons why high-fiber foods score so well in satiety. First, we eat them more slowly. Fiber increases chewing time. That means our bodies crank out more saliva and more gastric juices, which help to fill up our stomachs. Second, our body processes high-fiber foods more slowly than others, and nutrient absorption happens over a longer period. Both the stomach and the small intestine are kept busy longer and are less likely to start sending hunger signals until they're empty. This seems especially important at breakfast. Studies have found that the higher the fiber content of breakfast, the less food we take in later in the day. That's why I always recommend a high-fiber starch in the morning.

The bad news is that while the average person needs 25 to 35 grams per day of this magical stuff, most of us eat only 8 to 11 grams of fiber. Americans are missing a key point. Fiber matters—in fact, it's every dieter's best friend. Fiber consumption isn't just critical to health, it's one of the most important predictors of obesity. Dozens of studies have shown that overweight men and women have significantly lower fiber intake than men and women who maintain a healthy weight. So diets that banish fiber-rich foods not only hurt people's health in the long term, they set dieters up to fail and start the whole discouraging cycle all over again.

The Snack Factor Diet is loaded with fiber. My clients say the inclusion of fiber-rich foods is one of the best surprises about the plan. They wouldn't give them up for anything, whether it's a satisfying baked potato at lunch or a luscious mango for dessert. One word of warning, though. If you are currently eating a very low-fiber selection of foods, go slowly, and introduce high-fiber foods in small amounts. Some people say they get gas and diarrhea if they eat much more fiber than they are used to very quickly.

When you head to the store with your *Snack Factor* shopping list (see pages 229–31), bring your reading glasses. I'm going to ask you to read labels and check the number of fiber grams as often as possible. Let's start with crackers, one of my favorite snack foods, since they can satisfy both a salty and crunchy craving, and combine so beautifully with many proteins, like a wedge of creamy low-fat cheese or natural peanut butter.

A serving of Ritz crackers, for example—about five of them—has 80 calories, 4 grams of fat, and zero fiber. Reduced Fat Triscuits are a little better: a single serving (about seven crackers) has 120 calories, 3 grams of fat, and 3 grams of fiber. But a two-cracker serving of Kavli Hearty Thick Whole Grain Crispbread blows them both out of the water with 80 calories, zero grams of fat, and 4 grams of fiber. (Other favorites of mine include GG Scandinavian Bran Crispbread, with 16 calories and 3 grams of fiber, and FiberRich, with 40 calories and 5 grams of fiber.)

I promise: thirty minutes, sixty minutes, and even two hours from now, your stomach will still be giving the Kavli crackers the thumbs-up. With the Ritz? You'll be thinking about your next snack before you finish brushing the crumbs away. In terms of more bang for your calorie buck, those high-fiber crackers with cheese are the equivalent of finding an incredible designer handbag marked down to $20. What's not to love about that?

Finally, with all the fuss about fiber lately, many of my clients have asked me how I feel about faux fiber—the supplements you can take in pill or powdered form. The Snack Factor Diet will make sure you have enough fiber-rich foods that fiber supplements won't be needed. I would rather you get your fiber from food! If you have trouble getting in enough fiber or still have issues with constipation, fiber supplements *may* have a place in your diet, but I want you to focus first on foods! You'll be getting all your fiber attached to plenty of nutritious, tasty snacks and meals.

Having said that regarding supplements, it seems that there are more fiber-enriched food products in stores every day. I love these! Some are amazing. I especially love fiber-enriched yogurt, such as new Dannon Lite & Fit Crave Control, or a La Tortilla Factory tortilla with an impressive 14 grams in a single serving. That's almost a third of your day's requirement! What follows are some of my recommendations, but keep your eyes open and experiment—I'm sure you'll soon find favorites of your own.

FIBER ALL-STARS

In general, when looking for fiber-rich foods, I recommend foods that have at least 3 grams of fiber per serving. But there are some foods that are slightly lower in fiber but high in other benefits as well—like 2 cups of dark leafy greens, which pack an amazing amount of phytonutrients, with about 1 tablespoon (2 grams) of ground flaxseed, which is rich in omega-3 fats. Here are some of my favorite fiber-rich foods:

1 cup raspberries	8.0g
1 cup blackberries	7.6g
3 prunes	4.7g
1 small pear with skin	4.3g
2 dried figs	3.5g
1 medium orange	3.1g
1 cup mango	3.0g
1 small apple with skin	3.0g
1 kiwi	2.6g
1 small baked potato with skin	3.6g
½ cup corn	3.4g
¼ avocado	2.9g
1 medium carrot	2.3g
½ cup broccoli, asparagus	2.0g
1 small baked sweet potato	2.0g
1 medium tomato	1.5g
¼ cup chickpeas	3.5g
¼ cup kidney beans	2.8g
¼ cup black beans	2.5g
¼ cup black-eyed peas	2.0g

½ cup Fiber One cereal (contains artificial sweetener)	13.0g
⅓ cup Kellogg's All-Bran Extra Fiber	8.5g
¼ cup (uncooked) steel-cut oats	8.0g
½ cup Uncle Sam cereal	5.5g
½ cup cooked oatmeal	4.0g
5 GG Scandinavian Bran Crispbreads	15.0g
1 La Tortilla Factory Low-Carb/Low-Fat large size tortilla	14.0g
1 Thomas' Lite Whole Grain English Muffin	8.0g
1 KeriBar	5.0g
5 cups (air-popped) popcorn	5.0g
2 FiberRich crackers	5.0g
1 Dannon Light & Fit Crave Control	3.0g
1 slice 100% whole-grain wheat bread	2.0–6.0g

FACTOR THIS!

IS THERE SUCH A THING AS TOO MUCH FIBER?

Yes! A very high-fiber diet can rob your body of nutrients, so don't overdo it. And remember, fiber absorbs water as it travels through your digestive system—one more reason to make sure you're adequately hydrated.

THE SMARTEST CARBS

If all that mattered was fiber, we'd be content living on popcorn and oatmeal. But carbohydrates offer many other nutrients that are also very important. There are two main types of carbohydrates: starches (complex carbs such as pasta, bread, or rice) and sugars (simple carbs such as fruit, milk products, desserts, and candy).

Starches

The best breads, cereals, crackers, and pasta for us to eat, in terms of both providing the most nutrition and helping us to lose weight, are whole grains. Even though most Americans, on average, get only one serving of whole grains daily—which is what I recommend in the first month of the Snack Factor Diet—they're incredibly important. They give us the nutritional benefits of the entire grain: vitamins, minerals, dietary fiber, and other natural plant compounds called phytochemicals. All of these components play a role in the protection against cancer, heart disease, and diabetes.

Whole grains are made up of all parts of the grain: the bran (or fiber-rich outer layer), the endosperm (the middle part), and the germ (the nutrient-rich inner part). When grains are milled, or refined, the bran and germ portions are removed, leaving only the endosperm. This middle part of the grain is essentially empty carbohydrate calories. If we are going to consume the calories, why not benefit from the rest of the grain as well? Whole-grain foods contain all three layers, so you get the nutritional benefits of the entire grain.

Whole grains also seem to be essential to healthy weight loss. In the famous Harvard Nurse's Study, researchers found that the more high-fiber whole-grain foods women consumed, the less likely they were to be overweight. And the reverse was true as well: the more refined-grain foods they ate, the heavier they were. There is evidence that eating refined grains makes you crave more of them.

The biggest challenge in getting enough whole grains is

learning how to read labels correctly. A product that contains all whole grains (meaning that the whole grain is intact including the bran, germ, and endosperm) will be labeled "100% whole grain." Whole wheat flour is considered a whole grain, but *wheat flour* is not: *wheat flour* is simply a synonym for "flour"! In other words, it is the same white flour used to make that Duncan Hines cake you stayed away from! Often, breads, bagels, and pizza dough are called "wheat bread" or "wheat bagel," but they are really just made with some wheat flour and food coloring! This is not to say that there are *not* whole wheat bagels and whole wheat pizza out there; it just means that you need to know what to ask or look for. Look at both the ingredient list and the nutrition facts panel on any packaged food and try to choose foods that list whole grains.

FACTOR THIS!

100% WHOLE GRAIN?

The Whole Grains Council has come up with the Whole Grain Stamps to simplify packaging. The *100% Stamp* assures you that a food contains a full serving of whole grain in each labeled serving and that *all* of the grain is whole grain. The basic *Whole Grain Stamp* appears on products containing half a serving of whole grain per labeled serving. Note that not all products use the stamp.

Remember that the grain world encompasses much more than wheat. Other great whole grains include

amaranth
barley
brown rice

buckwheat
bulgur
corn
kamut
millet
oatmeal, whole or rolled oats
popcorn
quinoa
spelt
wild rice

Whole grains are available in various foods, from breakfast cereals to whole-grain pastas. You can even substitute whole-grain flours, including whole wheat and spelt for refined white flours when baking.

Sugars

Sugars are the most misunderstood carbohydrates. As soon as I say "sugar," most people envision candy, dessert, or soft drinks. But sugars are also a main component of fruits, vegetables, and dairy products—and I'm a big fan of all three. (Sometimes, my clients are surprised when I tell them that a single piece of fruit can contain 15 grams of sugar!)

A preference for sugar is something we are truly born with and seems to be part of our basic biological function. Most scientists agree that babies are born with the instinctive preference for sweets; it's an evolutionary adaptation from prehistoric times when food was scarce. Sugar implied calories, so our ancestors learned to seek out foods that tasted sweet, such as berries, knowing that they were a guaranteed source of energy.

So sugar does belong in our diet. But the problem is that Americans are way over the top in its consumption. Growing up in a culture where sugary foods are often given as rewards and/or seen as an indulgence, it's no wonder many Americans not only have a "sweet tooth" but also a whole mouth full of "sweet teeth"!

Over time, sugar has become available in more concentrated doses (as in the cookies and candy we indulge in a little too frequently). Sugar does occur naturally in milk and fruit, but it's the refined sugar, or sucrose, in the American diet that causes the greatest concern. On average, we eat 300 to 400 calories worth of refined sugar daily. That is thirty-one to forty-one pounds per year, and as a result, we have a distorted perception of how sweet many foods should be. And remember nutrient density? Get your sugar calories where they are needed most. Most of these 300 to 400 calories are nutrient-free.

So I urge my clients to really pay attention to the sugar they consume. When they're having it, I want them to make sure it's the healthiest kind of sugar, found in fruit and such dairy products as milk and yogurt. (For the first four weeks on Snack Factor, I will ask you not to eat any fruit. That's because it will help jump-start your weight loss and also lessen your appetite for sweet-tasting foods.)

Of course, every so often a client will say, "I can't give up these foods. I'm *addicted* to sugar." But that's simply not true, even given our natural preference for sweets. There's been no scientific evidence to show that sugar is addictive. Researchers agree that, unlike other established addictive substances, sugar does not cause uncontrollable cravings or lead to clinical withdrawal symptoms. A study on rats at Princeton University showed the possible existence of a sugar "dependency" resulting from extremely high levels of sugar consumption interspersed with periods of sugar deprivation. The study did not demonstrate the existence of a sugar addiction. But this sugar "dependency" may be why you feel sugar "highs" followed by sugar "lows." These highs and lows can disrupt sleep, cause increased consumption of calories, and lead to fatigue. As most of us know, sugar also has been proved to increase tooth decay. And who wants to be thin but tired and with a whole mouth full of rotten teeth? So the good news is that it's up to you: you really can control your intake of sugar. Don't blame your jellybean binges on an addiction!

The first step is to become aware of the sugar in the foods you eat, even those you consider to be "safe" diet choices, like yogurt. Use this as a guideline: a small piece of fruit has approximately 15 grams of sugar. Fruit is also natural and contains fiber—the nutrient density is high and the sugar is *not* added sugar. Obviously, 15 grams of sugar from candy is not even close to equivalent to what you find in fruit. But using the 15 grams as a guideline will help you to understand just how much is reasonable (provided you're getting nutrients as well). The worst sugar offender is HFCS—high fructose corn syrup. Read your food labels and steer clear of it.

FACTOR THIS!

I LIKE JUICE BETTER THAN FRUIT. IS THAT OKAY?

Actually, I'm sorry to say, no. The more we can eat whole fruits and vegetables, the better off we are. Juice contains some nutrients (although you'd be surprised at how little sometimes!) but not nearly as much fiber as the actual fruit. For example, an orange contains 70 calories, 7 grams of fiber, and 6 percent of your daily calcium. An 8-ounce glass of orange juice, on the other hand, has 110 calories, meets 2 percent of your daily calcium needs, and has practically no fiber. Which one sounds like a better deal to you? And when you can, include the skin on your fruits and vegetables to boost your fiber intake a little more. And for those days when you do decide to drink juice, make sure it's 100 percent juice, with no added sugar, and that you limit yourself to a single portion, which is 4 ounces.

THE MOST POWERFUL PROTEINS

After carbs, the next step is making sure you are eating the right kind of lean proteins. Moderately increasing the amount of lean meats and low or nonfat dairy products you consume will cause you to eat fewer calories overall and to lose weight.

Protein also has the most nutritional staying power. While the effect of simple carbs begins to wear off in thirty minutes or so, and complex carbohydrates after several hours, research has shown that even in a twenty-four-hour span, increased protein consumption increases satiety. And protein seems to be especially powerful in the morning, which is why I always recommend that clients start their day with a little, even if it's just a handful of nuts on breakfast cereal. Protein also modulates the rise and fall of blood sugar levels, keeping your energy supply on an even keel. That's why it's such a good idea to eat protein in combination with other foods, like adding a couple of teaspoons of almond butter to your morning toast. (You'll find that most of the snacks and meals I recommend contain at least a little bit of protein, for just that reason.)

If you like them, eggs are also a great morning protein source. Researchers at Saint Louis University found that women who started their day with an egg at breakfast not only ate less at lunch but consumed fewer calories in the course of the entire day.

Protein is also vital to health. Until we reach adulthood, it's critical for growth. After we're grown up, it is still important for tissue repair and to replace the hormones and enzymes our body uses in its many functions. It also acts as a backup energy source if carbohydrates are not available.

Keri's Favorite Lean Proteins

While there are many excellent lean meats and fish and meat substitutes (for more ideas see Chapter 5), this list encompasses some of my favorites. These lean choices are rich sources of protein and are either lower in calories and fat and/or excellent sources of omega-3s. Feel free to include your own favorites in your diet, too.

beef tenderloin
bison (buffalo)
chicken breast (no skin)
cod
egg whites
flounder
halibut
lobster
mussels
ostrich
pork tenderloin
salmon (wild)*
sardines (canned in water)
scallops
sea bass
shrimp
tofu
tuna (fresh or canned in water)
turkey breast (no skin)

* Salmon has more calories and fat per ounce than other foods listed here, but it is so rich in omega-3s that I have to include it on my favorites list. Remember, we want nutrient density.

The fattiest types of meat include marbled beef and lamb (marbling is the fat/cartilage in the meat), sausages, ground meats (not 95 percent lean), and dark poultry with the skin. If you are choosing a meat that is not from the lean-meat list, trim it of excess fat and remove any skin.

FANTASTIC FATS

Yes, there are good fats, even great fats. Healthy bodies need fat to function. And up to approximately one-third of the day's calories should come from fat, which plays so many crucial roles. Fat

- Helps us to burn fat
- Enables hormones to work properly
- Allows for the absorption of vitamins A, D, E, and K
- Insulates the body from the cold
- Protects organs
- Provides energy

But not all fats are our friends. On Snack Factor, the fats you choose will promote cardiovascular health. They include essential fatty acids, monounsaturated fats, and polyunsaturated fats. Saturated fats and trans fats (or hydrogenated fats) increase a person's risk for cardiovascular disease and heart attack, so they should be avoided as much as possible.

Heart-Healthy Fats	Food Sources	Cardiovascular Benefits
Monounsaturated fats	Olives, peanuts, flaxseeds and their oils, almonds, almond butter, canola oil, oil, avocado	Help increase "good" (HDL) cholesterol and decrease "bad" (LDL) cholesterol

Heart-Healthy Fats	Food Sources	Cardiovascular Benefits
Polyunsaturated fats	Corn oil, safflower oil, sunflower seeds and oil, sesame seeds and oil, soybeans (soy nuts, soy nut butter, and soybean oil), walnuts, pumpkin seeds, and tofu	Help reduce total cholesterol
Essential fatty acids, especially omega-3s	Fatty fish: salmon, albacore tuna, mackerel, trout, sardines, herring (flax, leafy greens, soybeans, walnuts, canola oil, and hemp oil are converted to EFAs in the body)	Reduce risk of developing blood clots, inflammatory disorders, cancer, heart disease, and high blood pressure; boosts metabolism to help weight-loss efforts

There are plenty of easy ways to incorporate these heart-healthy fats into your diet:

- Snack on a handful of almonds or other nuts instead of potato chips or other packaged fried foods.
- Substitute olive oil and other oil-based dressings for creamy salad dressings.
- Eat more fish! I recommend eating at least two servings of fish per week. Remember to stay away from the higher-mercury fish, including swordfish, shark, and tilefish.
- If you like vegetarian meals, like soy foods and tofu, try to have at least one or two vegetarian meals per week.

OMEGA-3S

Type and Portion Size	Amount of Omega-3
Land O'Lakes Fortified Egg (1 egg)	350mg
Flaxseed, ground (2 tbsp.)	3.51g
Walnuts (2 oz.)	2.27g
Uncle Sam Cereal (4 oz.)	1000mg
Silk Soy Enhanced Milk (8 oz.)	500mg
KeriBar (1 bar)	500mg
Smart Balance Light Spread (1 tbsp.)	300mg
Edamame (soybeans; 8 oz.)	1.03g
Smart Balance Omega Peanut Butter (1 tbsp.)	500mg
Wild Salmon (3 oz.)	1.8g
Sardines, canned (3 oz.)	1.3g

FACTOR THIS!

CRAZY ABOUT NUTS

For years, nuts have had a bad reputation because they are high in calories and fat. But they're making a big comeback, which thrills me. They're nutrition powerhouses, packed with protein and other "good for you" substances. If you choose raw nuts as opposed to salted nuts roasted in oil, you will reap the rewards from only "good" fats. And read the labels—avoid any fat that has the words *hydrogenated* or *partially hydrogenated* in it.

Here's the skinny on nuts:

- Most of the fats in nuts are unsaturated and may help increase your "good" cholesterol and lower your "bad" cholesterol.

- Walnuts are rich in omega-3s, which protect the heart and reduce inflammation.
- They're a good source of the antioxidant vitamin E and the B-vitamin folate, magnesium, calcium, and potassium.
- They're a good source of protein and fiber.
- Peanuts, walnuts, and hazelnuts are good sources of a certain amino acid known to help reduce blood pressure.
- Flavonoids found in nuts are a group of antioxidants that protect against heart disease and cancer.
- Nuts provide a great amount of satiety, which can help control your weight.

WHICH DAY IS THE BEST NUTRIENT BARGAIN?

MEAL PLAN A	MEAL PLAN B	The Skinny
Breakfast 1 slice white toast 1 tsp. butter 8 oz. 1% milk	**Breakfast** 8 oz. All-Bran Extra Fiber 1 tbsp. chopped walnuts 8 oz. skim milk	Portions similar, but in B you get fiber (All-Bran vs. white bread) and heart-healthy fat (walnuts vs. butter)
Snack 2 celery sticks 2 tsp. peanut butter	**Snack** 2 celery sticks 2 tsp. natural peanut butter	Same satisfaction to a craving, but in B you don't get the hydrogenated ("bad" fat) and added sugar found in many brands of peanut butter
Lunch Iceberg lettuce with celery and cucumbers 4 oz. steamed shrimp 2 tbsp. ranch dressing	**Lunch** Spinach salad with broccoli, celery, and cucumbers 4 oz. steamed shrimp ¼ avocado Balsamic and lemon dressing	Similar lunch, but in B you get more fiber, antioxidants, and omega-3 and none of the "bad" fat found in creamy salad dressings
Snack 1 Dannon Light & Fit Yogurt 10 almonds	**Snack** 1 FAGE Total 0% Yogurt 10 almonds	Both great choices! But if you have the option, I always recommend plain yogurt with no added sweetener

MEAL PLAN A	MEAL PLAN B	The Skinny
Dinner 4 oz. roasted chicken thigh and leg Steamed broccoli with 1 oz. Cheddar cheese Chopped salad with romaine lettuce, red onions, green peppers, and carrots Balsamic vinegar and lemon	**Dinner** 4 oz. roasted chicken breast (no skin) Steamed broccoli with 2 tsp. olive oil and garlic Chopped salad with romaine lettuce, red onions, green peppers, and carrots Balsamic vinegar and lemon	In B you get only lean protein (white meat) and heart-healthy fat (olive oil) vs. saturated fat (dark meat and Cheddar cheese)

So which meal plan is better?

Although both of these meal plans look good and seem to adhere to the Snack Factor Diet, Meal Plan B, packed with nutrient-dense foods, has less sugar and about one third the saturated fat as Meal Plan A, and eight times the omega-3 fats. Although the differences seem subtle (All-Bran versus white bread; spinach versus iceberg lettuce; avocado instead of creamy dressing), the extra punch of these few choices translates to four times the amount of fiber and much higher levels of the antioxidants (vitamins A, C, and E). *Plus, the foods in Meal Plan B provide more satiety because of the extra fiber and heart-healthy fats—which is one of the keys to the success of this diet!*

FACTOR THIS!

WHAT'S THE OPPOSITE OF NUTRIENT DENSE?

Many researchers would agree that foods rich in fats and sugar, but low in fiber and nutrition, are the polar opposite of nutrient-dense foods. The problem with these foods isn't just the fat and sugar. Swedish researchers

(continues)

have found that they disrupt the body's chemistry, blunting our satiety signals. We can just keep eating and eating and eating a hot fudge sundae, whereas halfway through an extra large salad, it's easier to say, "I've had enough."

FACTOR THIS!

SUPPLEMENT RECOMMENDATIONS

As I am sure you can tell by now, I am a big believer in getting nutrients through food. However, I do also recommend supplements—for insurance! You should still get your nutrients through food, and I never want to hear you say "I take calcium so I don't need to eat my yogurt!" If you choose to add supplements to your diet, here are a few of my favorites to start with:

Calcium

Daily recommended intake is 1,000 to 1,300 milligrams depending on age and gender. It is so important that if you do not feel you are getting 100 percent of your needs, you take a supplement. I recommend Rainbow Light Everyday Calcium with Enzymes: 4 tabs contain 1,200 milligrams calcium. Remember to split the milligrams throughout the day so you get approximately 300 to 600 at one time. This will help maximize absorption.

Omega-3*

Daily recommended intake is 650 milligrams (for DHA and EPA together). It is hard to get the amount of omega-3 we need from food to receive all of its benefits. Nordic Naturals Omega-3 or Carlson Super Omega-3 helps you get in adequate amounts. Two Nordic Natural tabs

* If you have trouble taking pills, Coromega is an orange- or orange-chocolate-flavored pudding-like texture that you can add to yogurt or yogurt shakes. One packet equals 650 mg total omega-3.

contain 220 mg DHA and 330 mg EPA; one Carlson tab contains 200 milligrams and 300 milligrams EPA.

Multivitamin

Mega Food Men's and Women's One Daily or New Chapter Men's and Women's One Daily are great choices because they are 100 percent whole-food based.

The point of all this nutrient density talk? You need carbohydrates. You need protein. You need fat. For health reasons *and* for weight-loss efforts, you need to maximize the nutrient density from all of the food you eat so you get the best carbohydrates, protein, and fat.

How Much Can You Eat?

What's Your Perfect Portion?

By now you're probably asking the most important question of all: what can I eat? After all, we can talk about protein, carbs, and fats all we want. But that's not much help when you stand in front of your fridge or read the menu at a restaurant. We don't walk into a steakhouse and order a serving of protein; we eat meat, which contains protein and some fat. Most people aren't able to be as specific as saying, "I'm craving carbs"; they're much more likely to say, "I feel like having pasta." We don't think of ourselves as stocking the fridge with calcium. We buy cheese and yogurt, which contain protein, carbs, and fat.

So portions—what you actually put on your plate—are where every aspect of this diet, whether HQ, nutrient density, or proportions, come together. Because I built my practice working with superbusy professionals, I wanted to make the Snack Factor Diet as simple as possible. I'm never (almost never) going to ask you to weigh your food; very few people have the time and patience to do that for more than a few days. (Of course, you can if you want to. But I suggest you find a better hobby.) Instead, use the general guidelines that follow for each type of food. Each set of general guidelines is followed by charts with specific portion sizes for packaged and branded foods. This list doesn't cover every imaginable food you'll encounter, but it does include many of my favorite nutrient-dense choices (and plenty to build weeks and weeks of menu plans around). Also, there are many other brands in stores today that are acceptable. To help you shop, I mention brands when a specific brand is a standout. For some foods, brand names are not as important, so I do not list them. The guidelines will help you to determine the portions of items that don't appear on the list.

Whenever I talk about a portion of something (as I will later in this chapter, when I outline your daily meal plans based on your weight), I'm referring to the portion sizes outlined here.

THE STARCH GROUP

NOTE: *All starch portions are listed from* highest fiber *option to* lower fiber *options—all are considered good options, but try to stick to the top of the list.*

Cereals
GENERIC PORTION
½ cup cereal

WHAT TO LOOK FOR
- Approximately 100 calories or fewer
- At least 5g fiber in cold cereal, 3g fiber in hot cereal
- No more than 6g sugar

WHAT DOES A PORTION LOOK LIKE?

A small fistful

KERI'S TIP

Measure cereal one time in a measuring cup. Try to use the same bowl every day so you remember what a portion looks like.

KERI'S PICK

Kellogg's All-Bran Extra Fiber (low-calorie, high-fiber, low-sugar) and Uncle Sam Instant Oatmeal with Whole Wheat Flakes & Flaxseed (portion-controlled packet; protein, fiber, and low-sugar)

BRAND AND PORTION SIZE

Kellogg's All-Bran Extra Fiber (½ cup)
Kashi Good Friends (¾ cup)
Nature's Path Flax Plus Flakes (¾ cup)
Nutritious Living Hi-Lo Original (½ cup)
Quaker Oat Bran Hot Cereal (⅔ cup, cooked)
Kashi GoLean (½ cup)
Uncle Sam Cereal (½ cup)
Nature's Path Optimum Slim (½ cup)
Kashi Heart to Heart (¾ cup)
Special K Low Carb Lifestyle Protein Plus (¾ cup)
Kellogg's Complete Wheat Bran Flakes (¾ cup)
Post Shredded Wheat 'n Bran (¾ cup)
Health Valley Organic Healthy Fiber Multigrain Flakes
    (¾ cup)
Steel-cut oats (¼ cup cooked)
Uncle Sam Instant Oatmeal with Whole Wheat Flakes &
    Flaxseed (1 packet)

Quaker Instant Oatmeal (1 packet) or regular oatmeal
(½ cup, cooked)

Waffles
GENERIC PORTION
1 waffle

WHAT TO LOOK FOR
- Approximately 100 calories or fewer
- Over 2g fiber
- No more than 3g fat

WHAT DOES A PORTION LOOK LIKE?
A "puffy" CD

KERI'S PICK
Both brands listed below are excellent choices if you are
craving a waffle! Better to eat home than in a restaurant because chances are a waffle in a restaurant is a much bigger
portion and much higher in fat and calories!
Kashi GoLean Waffles
Van's Multi Grain Waffles

Breads/Tortillas
GENERIC PORTION
1 slice bread, ½ pita, ½ English muffin, ½ roll or bun,
small tortilla

WHAT TO LOOK FOR
- Approximately 100 calories or fewer
- Over 2.5g fiber
- No more than 3g fat

WHAT DOES A PORTION LOOK LIKE?
A CD case

KERI'S PICK
Thomas' Light Multi Grain English Muffin (you can eat the whole muffin, and you get 8g of fiber, too) or La Tortilla Factory Low-Carb Tortilla

BRAND AND PORTION SIZE
Thomas' Light Multi Grain English Muffins (1 whole muffin)
La Tortilla Factory Low-Carb/Low-Fat Original Tortillas (1 tortilla)
Tumaro's Low in Carbs Multi Grain Tortillas (1 tortilla)
French Meadow Bakery Men's Bread (1 slice)
Thomas' Sahara Pita Wheat (½ pita)
Arnold Bakery Light Wheat Bread (2 slices)
Thomas' Hearty Grains Multi Grain English Muffins (½ muffin)

Crackers
GENERIC PORTION
Sorry. Because the size and makeup of crackers vary so dramatically, there isn't an exact number of crackers to make up a generic portion.

WHAT TO LOOK FOR
• Approximately 100 calories or fewer
• Over 3g fiber

WHAT DOES A PORTION LOOK LIKE?
Depends on size of crackers. Most important to look at calories and fiber.

Crackers are a great food source for fiber, so choose wisely and aim for the most fiber you can get.

GG Scandinavian Bran Crispbread (excellent source of fiber, and it's low calorie)—15g of fiber for 5 crackers (80 calories!)

NOTE: Kashi TLC crackers are lower in fiber, but make a good snack paired with hummus, reduced-fat cheese, or natural peanut butter.

BRAND AND PORTION SIZE
GG Scandinavian Bran Crispbread (5 crackers)
FiberRich Bran Crackers (2 crackers)
Wasa Fiber Rye [with Sesame and Oats] (2 crackers)
Ryvita Rye and Oat Bran Whole Grain Crispbread (2 crackers)
Kavli Hearty Thick Crispbread (2 crackers)
Dr. Kracker Klassic 3-Seed Flatbread (1 flatbread)
Kashi Original 7 Grain Crackers (7 crackers)

Chips and Stuff
GENERIC PORTION
Approximately 1 ounce (or less; see what to look for below)

WHAT TO LOOK FOR
- Approximately 100 calories or fewer
- At least 3g fiber per serving
- No more than 2g sugar

A big handful!

Most "chips" or chiplike products are high in calories even if they are the "healthy" version. Also, most do not contain much fiber or protein. Plus, they are very easily overeaten, and the bags they come in are usually more than one serving. It is very important to read labels here.

Glenny's Soy Chips are great if you are craving a salty crunchy snack and they are packed with soy protein!

BRAND AND PORTION SIZE
Jolly Time Healthy Pop Mini Bags (1 bag)
Bearitos Organic No Oil Added Microwave Popcorn (5 cups popped)
Glenny's Soy Chips (1 bag = 1.3 oz.)

Muffins
2-ounce muffin

• Approximately 100 calories or fewer
• Over 4g fiber
• No more than 2.5g fat

A child's fist or a small muffin top

KERI'S TIP

Most muffins have hidden fat, calories, and sugar. If you are eating a muffin, try to eat a packaged muffin that fits within the nutrition guidelines listed. Avoid all muffins/baked goods made with hydrogenated or trans fats.

KERI'S PICK

The Vitalicious VitaMuffin Sugar-Free/Low-Carb Velvety Chocolate Vitatop Muffin has fewer calories and more fiber than the other flavors, but note that it is made with sucralose.

BRAND AND PORTION SIZE

Vitalicious VitaMuffin (one 2-oz. muffin)

Vitalicious VitaMuffin Vitatop (one 2-oz. muffin)

Vitalicious All Natural Apple-BerryBran or Multi-Bran
   Vitatops

FACTOR THIS!

MY FAVORITE MUFFIN

This is my favorite way to indulge in a muffin! You can also make a few batches at a time and freeze them.

1¼ cups all-purpose flour

2 tablespoons sugar (see Note)

2 tablespoons ground flaxseeds

1 tablespoon baking powder

¼ teaspoon salt

2 cups Kellogg's All-Bran Cereal

1¼ cups skim milk

(continues)

2 egg whites
¼ cup chunky applesauce
1 teaspoon ground cinnamon

Preheat oven to 400°F.

Stir together flour, sugar, flaxseeds, baking powder, and salt. In separate large bowl, combine All-Bran and milk; let stand for 2 to 3 minutes. Add egg whites and applesauce, and mix well. Add flour mixture and stir until combined. Spoon into twelve 2½-inch muffin tins with liners. Bake for approximately 20 minutes. Dust with cinnamon and cool on rack. Serve.

12 servings

NOTE: The amount of sugar per serving is minimal, but you can substitute Splenda Sugar Blend for Baking (mix of Splenda and sugar) for the sugar in recipe.

Grains

GENERIC PORTION

⅓ cup cooked (unless otherwise specified)

WHAT TO LOOK FOR

- Approximately 100 calories or fewer
- Over 2g fiber
- Some protein

WHAT DOES A PORTION LOOK LIKE?

A mound the size of the top half of a hamburger bun

KERI'S PICK

Quinoa because it is a complete protein, meaning it contains all nine essential amino acids—something to boast about as a grain! And any whole wheat pasta with flaxseed!

BRAND AND PORTION SIZE

Bob's Red Mill Bulgur (⅓ cup, cooked)

Hodgson Mill Certified Organic Whole Wheat
  Gourmet Fettucine with Milled Flax Seed
  (½ cup, cooked)*

DeBoles Organic Whole Wheat Pasta (½ cup,
  cooked)

Ian's Whole Wheat Panko Breadcrumbs (¼ cup)

Kretschmer Wheat Germ (3 tablespoons)

Eden 100% Buckwheat Soba (½ cup, cooked)*

Kamut (⅓ cup, cooked)

Quinoa (⅓ cup, cooked)

Brown rice (⅓ cup, cooked)

Barilla Plus Pasta (½ cup, cooked)

Near East Long Grain and Wild Rice (⅓ cup,
  cooked)

Millet (⅓ cup, cooked)

Starchy Vegetables

GENERIC PORTION

½ to 1 cup

WHAT TO LOOK FOR

- Approximately 100 calories or fewer
- Over 2g fiber

WHAT DOES A PORTION LOOK LIKE?

Remember that mound similar to the top half of a hamburger bun?

* Contains omega-3!

Butternut squash because it has great flavor and is high in antioxidants and fiber.

TYPE AND PORTION SIZE
Butternut squash (1 cup, cooked)
Acorn squash (½ cup, cooked)
Peas (½ cup)
Yellow squash (1 cup, cooked)
Spaghetti squash (1 cup, cooked)
Zucchini (1 cup, cooked)
Sweet potato baked with skin (1 small)
Corn, frozen (½ cup)
Potato baked with skin (1 small)
Corn, ear (1 small)

Legumes
GENERIC PORTION
½ cup

WHAT TO LOOK FOR
- Approximately 120 calories or fewer
- Over 2g fiber
- Minimum 2 to 3 grams protein

WHAT DOES A PORTION LOOK LIKE?
That same mound similar to the top half of a hamburger bun

KERI'S PICK
Kidney beans—so easy to keep cans in your pantry and a great substitution for meat on a salad. And, of course, they are high in soluble fiber and folate and magnesium, all of which help protect your heart.

KERI'S TIPS

Beans are slightly higher in calories than the other starches mentioned above, but higher in fiber than most and a good source of protein.

The serving size of a legume may be different if you are using it as a starch versus as a lean protein. For example, if you add chickpeas to a salad as the main source of protein, versus when you also have chicken in your salad and add chickpeas as a starch. You will see what your portion of legumes as a lean protein is in Chapter 5.

TYPE AND PORTION SIZE

Split peas (½ cup)

Lentils (½ cup)

Black beans (½ cup)

Pinto beans (½ cup)

Chick peas (½ cup)

Kidney beans (½ cup)

White beans (cannellini beans) (½ cup)

Black-eyed peas (½ cup)

If choosing hummus, Tribe of Two Sheiks (2 tablespoons) is an excellent brand offering fewer calories than other commercial brands. For a bean soup, try Health Valley Fat Free Black Bean and Vegetable Soup (1 cup).

FACTOR THIS!

WHAT HAPPENED TO PASTA?

I admit it, pasta is one food I actively discourage people from eating, for two reasons. First, many of us grew up eating plates piled so high with spaghetti and meatballs that it's very difficult to reeducate ourselves

(continues)

about proper portion sizes. A one-pound box of angel-hair pasta, for example, is meant to serve eight people. Yet it's easy to eat a half pound of pasta in one "serving" and not even feel full. Which brings me to my second complaint. Conventional pasta—superhigh in carbohydrates yet very low in nutrition or fiber—is an empty food. So if you really crave pasta, try some of the many wonderful whole-grain pastas on the market. Their texture is a little chewier, but they do deliver valuable fiber and nutrients. But be careful to measure out portions before digging in. (Using the dry measure is easiest when you're at home, but in restaurants, the rule of thumb is that a single serving of pasta will look like half a baseball on your plate.) Many restaurants will allow you to order a half portion or appetizer-size portion of pasta for an entree. The best option is to look at pasta as your side dish and eat a lean protein as your main course. And of course, don't forget to fill up on vegetables so that you don't overdo the pasta!

VEGETABLES

GENERIC PORTION

One cup raw vegetables, ½ cup cooked vegetables, 2 cups lettuce—but don't be afraid to eat up as long as they're not cooked in fat! *I want you to fill up on vegetables. I never had a client not lose weight or gain weight from eating too much spinach!*

WHAT TO LOOK FOR

Color! I am a big fan of dark greens. But also veggies with rich colors such as red and orange are indicative of high nutrient density.

WHAT DOES A PORTION LOOK LIKE?

If you are eating greens, as I recommend at least two times per day, I want you to fill up on them. Fill your plate!

KERI'S TIP

Keep frozen vegetables around for fast, easy meals. Cascadian Farm organic frozen veggies are my favorite! Also, always order a steamed side dish of veggies when dining out—they will help fill you up.

KERI'S PICK

Like Popeye, I just can't get enough spinach—and neither can you.

NOTE: All vegetables listed are good sources of fiber and antioxidants. Vegetables with asterisks are slightly higher in calories. Remember, I want you to fill up on the greens as much as possible and use other vegetables for taste and variety.

TYPE

Acorn squash*
Alfalfa sprouts
Artichoke, boiled*
Artichoke hearts*
Arugula
Asparagus
Bamboo shoots
Bean sprouts
Beets*
Broccoli
Brussels sprouts
Cabbage
Carrots*
Cauliflower
Celery
Cherry tomatoes

Cucumber
Dandelion greens
Eggplant
Escarole
Green beans
Green onions/scallions
Hearts of palm
Iceberg lettuce
Jicama
Kale
Kombu seaweed noodles
Leeks
Mushrooms
Onion
Peppers (green)
Peppers (red)
Radish
Romaine lettuce
Sauerkraut
Snow peas
Spaghetti squash
Spinach, cooked
Spinach, raw
Summer squash
Swiss chard
Tomato†
Turnips
V8 Juice*
Water chestnuts*
Watercress
Zucchini

†For tomato sauce, try Colavita Marinara (½ cup). Look for up to 100 calories for ½ cup with less than 5 grams of sugar and no added sugar and oil.

THE MILK/YOGURT GROUP

GENERIC PORTION
6–8 ounces

WHAT TO LOOK FOR
- At least 5g protein
- No more than 15–20g sugar
- No more than 2.5g fat
- No more than 100 calories per serving

WHAT DOES A PORTION LOOK LIKE?
Check out a container of yogurt, or measure 1 cup of milk (you only have to measure this one time). Note that soy products are slightly higher in calories than milk or yogurt, but they are an excellent protein and calcium source, especially if you are vegan or lactose intolerant.

KERI'S TIP
Look for nonfat or low-fat options. Also, look for options with the most protein and/or added fiber. Read nutrient labels and avoid dairy products with high-fructose corn syrup.

KERI'S PICK
FAGE Total 0% Greek Yogurt is my favorite. It is low in sugar and calories and high in protein. And it tastes *delicious.* I also like Silk Soy Enhanced Milk because of the added omega-3s.

BRAND AND PORTION SIZE
DanActive Immunity Yogurt shakes (3.3 oz.)
Dannon Activa Yogurt (4 oz.)*

* Contains probiotics to help regulate digestive system.

Dannon Light & Fit With Crave Control (Splenda) (4 oz.)*
FAGE Total 0% Yogurt (5.3 oz.)
Friendship 1% Lowfat Cottage Cheese (4 oz.)
Lactaid 100 Skim Milk (1 cup)
Light n' Lively Cottage Cheese (4 oz.)
Silk Soymilk, Plain (8 oz.)
Silk Soymilk Enhanced (8 fl. oz.)
Silk Soy Yogurt (8 oz.)
Skim Plus Milk (8 oz.)†
Stonyfield Farm Light Yogurt (6 oz.)
Yoplait Smoothie Light (8 oz.)
Yoplait Light Yogurt (6 oz.)

LEAN PROTEINS (MEAT OR MEAT SUBSTITUTES)

GENERIC PORTION
Lean-protein portions vary based on your size:

- If you weigh less than 150 pounds, your protein portion is 3–4 ounces.
- If you weigh between 151 and 180 pounds, your protein portion is 4–6 ounces.
- If you weigh over 180 pounds, your protein portion is 6–8 ounces.

WHAT TO LOOK FOR
Low-fat choices (with the exception of salmon); in general, look for meat and poultry with less than 5–7 grams of fat per serving. Choose lean-meat sources—no skin, no marbling.

---

* Provides 3g fiber.
† Provides 40% calcium and 25% vitamin D.

WHAT DOES A PORTION LOOK LIKE?

Three to 4 ounces is approximately the size of the original iPod. If you get sliced meat from the deli counter, that's about 4 medium-thickness slices. And remember, if you are truly hungry at a meal, increase your veggie serving; then if you are still truly hungry, add a little protein. Your portion may end up being 5 ounces not 4; this does not mean you have "cheated" or been "bad." It just means you are listening to your HG.

KERI'S TIP

If you have a kitchen scale at home, weigh your lean meats *once* to visualize portions. I know I said you would not have to weigh your food, but just one time can be helpful for the future. I promise you won't have to do it again. If you purchase from a butcher or fish store, ask for a 4-ounce portion. Choose fish at least two times per week.

KERI'S LEAN PROTEIN PICK

I love scallops and cod! Also, see my full list of favorites on pages 88–89.

NOTE: Pregnant women should avoid swordfish, king mackerel, tilefish, tuna, and shark owing to high mercury levels.

For protein foods, use the list below and you will be guided on the appropriate portion in Chapter 5, based on your calorie needs.

Poultry
TYPE
Chicken
Cornish hen
Turkey

BRANDS
Applegate Farms Organic Roasted Chicken (deli slices)
Applegate Farms Organic Roasted Turkey (deli slices)
Bell and Evans Fully Cooked Grilled Chicken Breasts
Purdue Short Cuts
Shady Brook Farms Turkey Breast 93% Lean Ground
SnackMasters Natural Range Grown Jerky (1 oz.)

Fish
Clams
Cod
Flounder
Halibut
Imitation crab (surimi)
King Crab
Lobster
Mahimahi
Mussels
Red snapper
Salmon, wild
Scallops, large sea
Shrimp (fresh)
Shrimp in bag (frozen)
Sole
Swordfish
Trout
Tuna, bluefin, raw
Tuna, canned in water (chunk light)
Tuna, fresh, cooked

BRANDS
Blue Hill Bay Baked Salmon with Cracked Pepper
EcoFish Frozen Shrimp

EcoFish Salmon Fillet (frozen)
King Oscar Sardines, packed in water
SnackMasters Natural Ahi Tuna Jerky
SnackMasters Natural Salmon Jerky
Starkist Albacore Lemon and Cracked Pepper Tuna Fillets
Starkist Light Meat Tuna Fillets
Whole Foods Whole Catch Wild Alaskan Sockeye Salmon
   Fillets (frozen)

Game
TYPE
Bison (buffalo) burger or steak
Ostrich
Venison

BRANDS
Blackwing Organic Jerky
Blackwing Ostrich Burger
Trader Joe's Ostrich Steak

Eggs
Egg (omega-3 fortified is best)

BRANDS
Egg Creations Egg Substitute
Eggology 100% Egg Whites
Papetti's All Whites 100% Liquid Egg Whites
Papetti's Better 'n' Eggs Plus

Hot Dogs and Sausages
BRANDS
Applegate Farms Chicken Hot Dog
Applegate Farms Organic Chicken & Apple Sausage

Applegate Farms Turkey Hot Dog
Han's All Natural Chicken or Turkey Sausage

Meat
Beef, 95% lean ground
Beef, Sirloin
Beef, T-bone
Beef tenderloin
Ham, extra-lean
Lamb Loin
Pork, center loin chops
Pork, cutlet
Pork, tenderloin
Veal, loin

BRANDS
Applegate Farms Organic Sliced Roast Beef
Oh Boy! Oberto Beef Jerky

Soy Products
BRANDS
Seapoint Farms Edamame
Woodstock Farms Firm Tofu

Legumes
BRANDS
Health Valley Fat Free Black Bean and Vegetable Soup

TYPES
Black beans
Black-eyed peas
Chickpeas
Kidney beans

Lentils
Pinto beans
Split peas
White beans (cannellini beans)

Cheese
TYPES
Cottage cheese, low-fat or nonfat
Feta cheese
Mozzarella
Other reduced-fat cheeses

FATS

GENERIC PORTION
1 slice cheese = 1 ounce = 1-inch cube or CD or 2 teaspoons nut spreads

WHAT TO LOOK FOR
Healthy fat and healthy fat only. No added hydrogenated or partially hydrogenated oils or trans fats. For example, when choosing peanut butter, go for brands that list only peanuts in the ingredients list, and do not include any hydrogenated oils.

KERI'S TIPS
Again, choose healthy fats when picking your fat portions—avocado, olive oil, nuts, flaxseed, for example. And remember, cheese is not a "healthy" fat, but it does contain calcium, so in moderation it is an absolutely fine choice. The recommendations I make are for reduced-fat versions of cheese, so you get the benefits without the drawbacks.

"Reduced fat" often means increased sodium, so be sure to

read the entire nutrition facts panel. Substitute plain low-fat yogurt and Dijon mustard for mayonnaise in tuna, chicken, and salmon salad.

Choose a sharp-flavored cheese. You'll need less of it to get a whole lot of flavor!

Oils and Dressings

TYPE AND PORTION SIZES
Canola oil (2 tsp.)
Corn oil (2 tsp.)
Olive oil (2 tsp.)
Safflower oil (2 tsp.)
Salad dressing, oil-based (1 tbsp.)
Sunflower oil (2 tsp.)

BRANDS
Keri's Lemon Dressing (1 tbsp.)

Nuts and Seeds

PORTION SIZES
Almonds (10, or 1 tbsp. chopped)
Flaxseeds, ground meal (2 tbsp.)
Hazlenuts (8)
Peanuts (15)
Pecan halves (8)
Pine nuts (1 tbsp.)
Pumpkin seeds (1 tbsp.)
Soy nuts (1 tbsp.)
Walnut halves (7 or 1 tbsp. chopped)

BRANDS
Arrowhead Mills Natural Peanut Butter (2 tsp.)
I. M. Healthy Soy Nut Butter (2 tsp.)
Smuckers Natural Peanut Butter (2 tsp.)

Olives and Cheese

PORTION SIZES

American cheese (1 slice)*

Avocado (¼ of medium)

Olives, large (12)

Olives, small (17)

Parmesan cheese, grated (3 tbsp.)

BRANDS

Alpine Lace Reduced Sodium Muenster Cheese (1 slice)

Alpine Lace Swiss Cheese (1 slice)

Athenos Feta, Crumbled (2 oz.)

Athenos Feta, reduced-fat (2 oz.)

Baby Bell Light Cheese (1 piece)

Cabot Cheddar 50% Light (1-oz. cube)

Friendship Farmer Cheese (2 tbsp.)

Goat Cheese (1 oz.)

Horizon Organic Shredded Part-Skim Mozzarella Cheese
(2 oz.)

Kraft Crumbles Low-Moisture Part-Skim Mozzarella Cheese
(2 oz.)

Laughing Cow Light Cheeses (2 wedges)

Organic Valley Stringles Part-Skim Mozzarella Cheese (1)

Eggs

BRANDS AND PORTION SIZES

Country Hen Organic Eggs with Omega 3 (1 extra-
large egg)

Horizon Organic Egg (1 egg)

Land O'Lakes All-Natural Eggs with Omega 3 (1 large egg)

* Note higher fat.

FRUIT

NOTE: After the first month on the diet, you will add a fruit portion.

GENERIC PORTION
1 small fruit or 1 cup cubes or berries

WHAT DOES A PORTION LOOK LIKE?
Tennis ball

KERI'S TIPS
Go for fresh, in-season fruit as often as possible. Avoid juice and dried fruit. (I do have dried fruit in some of the snacks in Chapter 5; however, it is used in portion control and with protein or fat to minimize the effect on blood sugar. If you can't control yourself, stay away altogether. Also, never have dried fruit with added sugar.)

KERI'S PICK
Berries are my favorite. They are high in antioxidants, fiber, and flavor.

NOTE: *All fruits are listed from* highest fiber *option to* lower fiber *option—all are considered good choices.*

TYPE AND PORTION SIZE
Raspberries (1 cup)
Blackberries (1 cup)
Passion fruit (3 medium)
Pear (1 small)
Blueberries (1 cup)
Orange (1 medium)

Strawberries, sliced (1 cup)

Figs (2 medium)

Apricot, dried (9 halves)

Papaya (1 cup)

Banana (1 small)

Apple (1 small)

Apricot, fresh (3 small)

Kiwi (1)

Mixed fruit cup (1 cup fresh fruit)

Pineapple (1 cup)

Peach (1 medium)

Santa Cruz Organic Apple Sauce (4 oz. container)

Mango (½ medium)

Plum (1 large fruit)

Cherries (½ cup)

Prunes (3)

Cantaloupe (1 cup)

Honeydew (1 cup)

Grapefruit (½ fruit)

Seedless grapes (15)

Watermelon (1 cup)

Del Monte fruit cups packed in water (4 oz. container)

Pomegranate (½ medium)

Tropicana Fruit pop (1 bar)

FACTOR THIS!

PORTION DISTORTION

Just reading these lists probably gave you a little wake-up call about portion sizes. And no wonder, since so many of us have a very unrealistic—

(continues)

not to mention unhealthy—sense of portion control. After all, we live in a country where the Olive Garden, which features all-you-can-eat pasta along with unlimited garlic bread, is one of the most popular restaurant chains. But even upscale restaurants serve much more food than we should eat. (Restaurant portions have gotten so out of control that the Food and Drug Administration is asking restaurants to limit their portion sizes!)

Since you're reading this book, I'm willing to bet you fall into one of three portion personalities:

1. You're virtuous and strict with your portions at mealtimes. But when it comes to less structured eating—like chips and dip at a party—you find it difficult to track how much you're actually eating.
2. You have a good sense of what healthy portions of any given food are, but you never follow them. For you, *portion* is an ugly word, like *budget.* It's got a stingy, controlling ring to it.
3. You're so confused that you have no idea what portions are what.

Whichever type you are, adjusting to the Snack Factor portions, while not effortless, is far easier than most people imagine it will be. The real key to figuring out your ideal portion size is as simple as measuring your HQ. No matter what you may be eating, you must stop when your HQ reaches 4—that "I feel satisfied with not one bit of fullness, and I don't feel gross leaving the table!" feeling. (Remember, on the HQ scale, a 1 means you're as stuffed as if it were just after overindulging in a Thanksgiving dinner, while a 10 means that you're hungry enough to snack on the centerpiece.)

That means you don't just have to ask yourself, "How hungry am I?" when you sit down to a meal, but also as the meal progresses. Be patient: I am asking you to re-learn the concept of hunger. And that's not easy, because so many of us have appetites that are bigger than our actual hunger.

It's important to eat *slowly*. By making each meal and snack last a little longer, you're giving your body a huge physiological advantage. That's because both hunger and satiety are governed by a complex set of hormonal responses. Ghrelin, for example, is a hormone we secrete that tells our brains that we're hungry. Leptin is a hormone we manufacture in our fat cells that tells our brains to stop eating because we've had enough. But that process doesn't happen in a few minutes—which, unfortunately, is how fast some of us can polish off three helpings of angel hair primavera. It can take up to twenty minutes for digestive hormones and our brains to get their signals straight.

My clients have all had lots of success with these little tricks for making a meal last longer:

- Putting their forks down between bites
- Sipping water between bites
- Engaging in conversation
- Shutting off the TV if they're eating alone
- Sitting down to the table instead of hunching over the sink or standing in front of the fridge

I know these tips may seem silly. And they will definitely feel a little foreign when you first try them. But they are actually very powerful. If you practice, they'll become a habit that can take off an average of 100 calories per meal (that's about three fewer bites)!

It also helps to know that in some foods, portion size matters—a lot. When it comes to fat and starch foods (and of course, sweets and alcohol), it's easy to overdo it. So with these foods, portion control really counts. Remember, you can—and I want you to!—include these foods in your life. But since they are so easily overeaten, it's easy to pile on the calories long before your satiety hormones have the chance to kick in, and before your brain notices that your HQ has shifted a notch or two.

In other foods, portions don't matter at all. There are many foods that you can eat as much of as you want to. For example, although it may be important to limit yourself to just 2 teaspoons of oil or 1 tablespoon of dressing, it's fine to pour on the vinegar and enjoy another helping (or two or three) of salad. (Check out the pour-them-on condiments on page 102.) Sure, these foods do contain some calories. But celery, cucumbers, lettuces, spinach, and asparagus are so high on flavor, texture, and phytonutrients that it's safe to say you can eat a lot and still be calorically controlled. When my clients ask me what size portion of vegetables they should have, I tell them to knock themselves out.

FACTOR THIS!

WHEN IN DOUBT, EAT VEGETABLES.

Still hungry? Eat your veggies and protein. There are times, particularly when you're just starting, when you're going to feel a little confused about what to do next. Your HQ will alert you that you are still hungry. I always suggest that clients have another serving of vegetables, and then see how they feel. Still hungry? Then go for another few bites of your lean protein.

Now, think back on all the times when you went back for seconds,

and maybe even thirds, of high-carb, high-fat foods like mashed potatoes and gravy. Isn't it empowering to realize that probably a few bites
more of a good lean protein would have satisfied you, whereas an extra
three servings of macaroni and cheese wouldn't do the trick?

Sometimes clients ask me about those "bad" vegetables,
like beets and carrots, that contain higher amounts of sugar. I
tell people to relax. No, these aren't what I call "free" foods,
in that you shouldn't eat them endlessly. But I promise that
America is not having an obesity epidemic because people are
overeating carrots. So enjoy.

MAKING PORTIONS A HABIT

Once you get into the Snack Factor mind-set, these portions
will feel like second nature. I promise, you're going to learn to
love the way your body feels with an HQ of 4. Your energy
level will be up, you'll feel calm and focused, and you just
won't want to feel any fuller than that. Until then, I'm going to
ask you to make some straightforward changes in your behavior that will help you make this portioning a healthy habit:

- Like a Boy or Girl Scout, you need to be prepared. Make
  sure your refrigerator is always stocked with the kinds of
  vegetables you like to nosh on. Cucumbers, celery, pre-
  bagged salads, presliced mushrooms, and peppers all can
  save you time and make pulling together a salad effortless
  instead of like an evening with Emeril.

- Go ahead, and ruin your appetite. I know, your mother always told you not to eat too soon before a meal, but I'm

here to tell you: having a healthy snack before any eating occasion, whether it's going out for dinner or to a big family eating extravaganza, will help you stay more in control of the portions you choose.

- Experiment. We need variety to satisfy us just as much as we need food to fill us up. Let's say you're having a grilled chicken breast with steamed spinach for dinner, and maybe—because you're not the most inventive cook, and besides, you're busy! —that's what you had last night. Turning it into a simple but satisfying chicken Parmesan, with a tomato sauce and sprinkled Parmesan cheese, will make the dinner feel much more satisfying to you than a rerun of last night's steamed spinach. That's one reason I'm such a big fan of frozen vegetables and simple condiments and spices: it's easier to stock up on an appealing and intriguing variety of vegetables without worrying about spoilage. Sometimes, clients will neglect this rule about variety, and inevitably it sets them up for failure. I promise, even if you're the kind of person who gets pretty comfortable in a food rut, after three nights of grilled chicken and spinach, you're setting yourself up for a major boredom binge. Challenge yourself: buy two new vegetables every time you hit the supermarket.

- Make individual portions ahead of time. Measure out single servings of almonds or walnuts in Ziploc bags to put in your briefcase or gym bag. Prepack vegetable assortments in the fridge so you can bring them to nibble on in the car. Buy KeriBars or other healthy snack bars and store them at the office. The idea is to make grabbing the right-size portion as effortless as possible.

- Snack often enough to keep your HQ between 4 and 6. Nothing sets you up for overeating more than letting yourself get too hungry. When you're ravenous, it's only natural to tear into a meal as if there's no tomorrow, without taking a break to listen to your body tell you when you've had enough.

- Always portion out your meals before you sit down to eat. Serving foods family style—with a big serving dish on the table—makes it too easy to just habitually reach for seconds. Even that little walk back into the kitchen will give your HQ a better chance to kick in and reassess whether you need seconds or not.

- In restaurants, take the offensive. Get used to the idea that when it comes to portions, most of America has lost its mind. I always suggest that clients check out a restaurant's menu ahead of time if they can (thanks to the Internet, many restaurants allow you to do this). Offer to share an entree, or at least, cut yours in half as soon as it arrives, and bag the rest. And don't be afraid to ask for the little changes that make your life easier. Ask the waiter not to bring the breadbasket or the chips, for example; if your dining companions want them, set them on the other side of the table.

- When eating out, treat yourself to a side order of different steamed vegetables. Add garlic or lemon, or sprinkle on sea salt. Unfortunately, when you order vegetables sautéed (even "lightly"), they often come drenched in oil. Vegetables add variety, make the meal more interesting, and help fill you up!

A NOTE ABOUT CONDIMENTS

Here are some of my favorite condiments. They add flavor and can easily allow you to add variety and creativity to some of your favorite dishes.

POUR-THEM-ON CONDIMENTS
(USE AS MUCH AS YOU LIKE OF THESE!)

Dijon mustard

Spicy brown mustard

Salsa (I love Walnut Acres Midnight Sun Salsa)

Vinegar (red wine, white wine, balsamic, cider, fig, raspberry)

Hot sauce

Lemon or lime juice (True Lemon/True Lime; see www.truelemon.com)

Tabasco sauce

Soy sauce (reduced sodium)

Pickle relish

Wishbone Salad Spritzers

COOKING SPRAYS

Spectrum Extra Virgin Olive Oil, and Canola Oil

Mazola Pure Olive Oil, Canola, and Butter Flavor

I recommend that you stick to the above condiments as well as include herbs and spices. When you have to have the ketchup on your lean burger, there is no harm in having a portion. Aim to have one portion of the condiment you choose below and not simply pile it on. Also, do not indulge in these more than once a day.

PORTIONED CONDIMENTS

Worcestershire Sauce—2 tablespoons

Heinz Organic Ketchup—2 tablespoons

Polaner All Fruit—1 tablespoon

Smucker's Simply 100% Fruit—1 tablespoon

Polaner Sugar Free (Splenda)—1 tablespoon

HIGH-SUGAR CONDIMENTS

Barbeque sauce—1 tablespoon

Duck sauce—1 tablespoon

Teriyaki sauce—1 tablespoon

Honey mustard—1 tablespoon

Cocktail sauce—¼ cup

SALAD DRESSINGS

Vinegars, lemon juice, mustard, and soy sauce—all in different combinations—make excellent low-calorie and low-fat dressings. Experiment!

Keri's Lemon Dressing (1 tablespoon)

½ cup extra-virgin olive oil

¼ cup fresh lemon juice

½ teaspoon salt

¼ teaspoon freshly ground black pepper

Dijon Vinaigrette

⅓ cup water

¼ cup white wine vinegar

1 tablespoon Dijon mustard

Salt and pepper to taste

½ packet of Splenda (if a sweeter dressing is desired)

Yogurt Herb Dressing (use 2 tablespoons as a condiment serving)

1 cup nonfat plain yogurt

1 tablespoon Dijon mustard

2 tablespoons chopped chives

2 tablespoons fresh lemon juice

HERBS AND SPICES

Herbs are an excellent addition to many recipes and foods; they lend a variety of delicious flavors to foods you might not otherwise be enticed by in your pre–Snack Factor days. Try using a mixture of chopped fresh herbs or dried herbs to marinate fish, poultry, and meat, or sprinkle herbs such as rosemary or thyme on your vegetables and roast them. Garlic not only adds flavor but also has health benefits, including antioxidant properties. Cinnamon is a wonderful addition to yogurt or cottage cheese, and also has potential health benefits, including helping control blood sugar levels and cholesterol levels. Look for herbs that are in season and aim to use those on your foods, but also keep jarred herbs and spices around so they are always accessible.

In the next chapter, you will synthesize all of the information you've gleaned so far about snacking, nutrient density, HQ and food timing, proportions, and now portions to start the Snack Factor Diet!

The Snack Factor Diet

The First Four Weeks and Beyond

Now that you know just how much snacking can help you lose weight, and you know everything there is to know about your HQ, proportions, nutrient density, and portions, let's get started on the diet.

First, let's get real. I know that if you're reading this book, chances are good that this isn't your first stab at losing weight. I'm betting you've got plenty of what I call "dieting assets," even if you don't think of them that way. Maybe you already like to exercise and drink plenty of water, or have the kind of job that makes planning regular gym visits easy. But you've probably also got some dieting baggage: those stubborn habits that have sabotaged your weight-loss efforts before.

I think of them as Nine Diet Traps from Hell. And while you may think you're unique in your struggle, I promise that the challenges are *very* common and painfully predictable. And I'm here to tell you that, yes, there is a way out. For the

next three days, just try your best to make the changes sug-
gested (following each trap). In three days, you can break
your bad diet habits forever!

Don't expect to do everything perfectly, or even all that
well. Like all habits, they're behaviors so deeply ingrained in
your daily routines that you often don't see how much they
control your eating. Three days will be enough to give you a
clear sense of where you're strongest, as well as a sense of the
baggage you're ready to ditch. And within thirty days, these
life-changing routines will be so well established that they'll
begin to feel as if you've been eating in this healthy pattern
your whole life.

Addressing these nine diet traps—with patience and
consistency—will set you up to win. You'll keep your metabolism revved, enabling you to lose weight painlessly while
maintaining your high energy levels. Even in these early days,
success feeds on success: because you're feeling good, it's easier to make healthy food choices. Already the sugar cravings
start to subside. And you gain the confidence you need to see
that, yes, you *can* get off the dieting roller coaster forever.
And building on the healthy foundation you're creating with
these nine new habits, you're going to be able to achieve and
maintain a healthy weight, without ever feeling hungry again.

You'll start to realize that the Snack Factor Diet isn't my
diet. It's *your* diet, a 100 percent original. Sure, I'll help you
create the framework, but what and when you eat will be entirely up to you. Because you're creating the plan, which I'll
teach you to tweak through trial and error, it will be much
easier to stick with it. Soon it won't feel like a diet at all—simply
the way you choose to eat. But first, let's get those traps out
of the way.

THE NINE DIET TRAPS FROM HELL— AND HOW TO OVERCOME THEM!

Diet Trap 1: Mindless Eating

Many of us nibble all the time, and often we have a pretty distorted idea of how much we actually eat—or don't eat—in any given day.

FOR THE NEXT THREE DAYS

Start a food journal. You'll find the form I like best on pages 232–33. Or you can download them at *www.snack factordiet.com*. Don't worry—you won't be writing a food journal forever! When it comes to making meaningful life changes, researchers have found that simple journals make a big difference in actually changing habits. I see it work every day in my practice. Make yourself do it.

Diet Trap 2: Ignoring Your HQ

Everything in this book—and everything I tell my clients—is based on this essential principle. It's so important that I've set aside all of Chapter 3 to help you fully understand why this little secret—a number on a scale of 1 (stuffed) to 10 (famished)—is all that stands between you and that favorite dress or pair of 34-inch slacks you've got hanging *way* in the back of your closet. It's a question you need to ask yourself every time you get ready to eat, whether it's a balanced meal you've lovingly prepared for yourself, a romantic night at your favorite restaurant, or a bag of greasy popcorn you snagged at the corner deli. *How hungry am I?* Don't believe me? HQ is so important that it's all I ask my private clients to do for the first week. And most of them lose weight without making a single other change.

FOR THE NEXT THREE DAYS

Record your HQ in your food journal before every meal and snack, either using the forms on pages 232–33 in this book, from my Web site, or just jotting it down in your daily calendar. After thirty days, you'll have learned how to manage your eating so that you are seldom hungrier than a 6 ("I guess I am about ready to eat" or more full than a 4 ("I feel satisfied, with not one bit of fullness").

Diet Trap 3: Neglecting Your Water Intake

Yes, I know you know that eight glasses a day are essential for healthy weight management. In fact, if you had a dollar for every time someone told you that, you'd probably have *two* houses in the Hamptons by now. But for many people who struggle with their weight, it's not just the number 8 that's magic, it's *when* you drink them. In other words, simply drinking a liter of Evian after you get home from work is missing (half) the point.

FOR THE NEXT THREE DAYS

Start each morning with a big glass of water. (I recommend squeezing fresh lemon juice into it.) I teach my clients to carry packets of True Lemon travel packets in their purse or briefcase. Lemon water helps many people feel good about drinking water, and some experts think lemons may help the liver and other major organs function better. In Ayurvedic medicine, lemon juice in warm (or even hot) water is thought to cleanse and tone the liver, and nutrition researchers believe that the phytochemicals in the skin of the lemon may help prevent certain cancers. With or without lemon, drink one glass of water before each meal and one glass during each meal.

Diet Trap 4: Black-and-White Eating

We've all been there: at 4:00 P.M. you're so hungry you pounce on the brownies that a well-meaning coworker brought to work. (Don't you *hate* those people?). That night, when the waitress comes around with the bread basket before dinner, you dive into that, too. "I already ate the brownies," you think. "My whole diet day is shot." With that kind of thinking, it's just too easy to order the pasta in cream sauce, then dessert, and tell yourself you'll start your diet all over again in the morning. Or next Monday. Or after you finally finish that enormous project at work.

FOR THE NEXT THREE DAYS

While breaking out of this black-and-white way of thinking is hard, I promise you that eating is much more fun in the world of living color! So you had the brownies—big deal! So you had some bread and butter—who cares? So you had three helpings of brown rice instead of one. Don't turn it into an excuse for a three-day binge of eating whatever you feel like. Remind yourself that every meal is a clean slate. *Every meal or snack is an opportunity to eat healthy foods.* Every day is "Monday morning"—a chance to start fresh, to give your body the nutritious food it deserves and give you the waistline you want. And give up on the idea of a penance meal. Just because you overdid it earlier in the day, that doesn't mean you have to punish yourself with a bone-dry salad or a boring little piece of grilled chicken. Each meal is a new beginning: make it healthful, well balanced, and inviting. By thinking this way, you will end up eating a more balanced and a less caloric diet throughout the week.

Diet Trap 5: Watching the Scale Too Closely

Some people are so obsessed with losing weight that they jump on and off the scale constantly, crushed or elated with every little fluctuation. Meaningful weight loss happens relatively slowly—about ten pounds a month if you follow this plan—and it builds up over time. If you watch it too closely—if the scale doesn't budge after a weekend when you feel like you were a saint, or worse, goes up a pound—you just feel like giving up and having a piece of chocolate cake.

FOR THE NEXT THREE DAYS

Don't weigh yourself until the third day. In fact, I recommend that most of my clients weigh themselves once a week (and if you've had a long tumultuous relationship with food and the scale, it's fine to toss the scale and go by the way your clothes fit). It's also helpful to figure out what physicians consider to be a more meaningful number: your body mass index, or BMI. The BMI is a measure that adjusts body weight for height. You can calculate yours by going to http://nhlbi support.com/bmi/. A healthy weight for adults is defined as a BMI of from 18.5 to less than 25; overweight as greater than or equal to a BMI of 25; and obese as greater than or equal to a BMI of 30. That means that a 5-foot-4-inch woman who weighs 155 pounds has a BMI of 26.6, which is above the healthy range.

Weight-loss experts find the BMI approach beneficial because it is often a better indicator of risk for the diseases associated with obesity. Yes, at 155 pounds the woman in this example *is* overweight—there's no waffling about that. But BMI is also more forgiving than the old "ideal body weight" concept, which said that a 5-foot-4-inch woman, ideally, should weight 120 pounds. Using the BMI, this woman is in a healthy range if her weight is anywhere from 108 to 145 pounds. Also remember, numbers—whether your BMI or what's on your scale—aren't the be-all and end-all. For example, a bodybuilder may have a BMI that makes him "obese" because of his high muscle percentage. Use the numbers as guidelines. I ask my clients "When did you feel your best?" "How much did you weigh then?" Often your own numbers, not the numbers put out by the government, are the best guidelines.

Follow this plan with *patience* and *consistency*, and the weight will come off. Here's a classic example: A client will start with me, and let's say she weighs 156 pounds. Within the first week, she's lost three pounds. She's elated, but then she has a "bad" weekend—maybe she ate too much salty food, or it's very hot and she's bloating, or she's premenstrual. She gets on the scale and it says 156 again, and she's crushed. I've heard clients wail: "I weigh the same as when I started!"

But that's not true, and it's so important to keep in mind that everybody's weight fluctuates several pounds. At any point within a day or two of starting the diet, she might have weighed 156 to 160. I just happened to weigh her in when she was at the low end. And after a week of following Snack Factor, her range was more likely 152 to 156. So she actually shifted into a lower range, but the scale doesn't measure that. That's why it's so important not to get bogged down by the scale. How do you feel? Do you have enough energy? Are you sleeping well? Are you feeling calm? How does your body feel—are your jeans a little looser? Can you see a little more collarbone? Those changes are often far more meaningful than any old numbers.

Diet Trap 6: Skipping Breakfast

Just when I think I've heard every possible excuse in the world from clients—why they're too busy, just not hungry that early, don't like breakfast foods, or eating too early makes them overeat the rest of the day—a new one comes along. (For nutritionists like me, these excuses are the equivalent of "The dog ate my homework" or "The check is in the mail"!)

No more excuses. Researchers have figured out that dieters who *eat* breakfast lose significantly more weight over a twelve-week period than those who *skip* breakfast. If you're still not convinced, it's worth pointing out that one of the traits that distinguishes successful dieters—those people who have lost at least 10 percent of their body weight and kept it off for more than a year, and are part of the National Weight Control Register—is that they eat a healthy breakfast each day.

Often, breakfast-skipping clients tell me they hate to eat breakfast because it makes them hungrier at lunch. "Great!" I say. "That means your metabolism is working. And if you're hungry at lunch, then eat!"

FOR THE NEXT THREE DAYS

Eat breakfast, and—this is the only instance you'll hear me suggest this—eat even if you aren't hungry. It doesn't have to be elaborate or involve any cooking—not even a microwave. A good nutrition bar, a drinkable yogurt, a hard-cooked egg or peanut butter on fiber crackers are all easy choices. Pay attention to how hungry you are and how you feel afterward.

Diet Trap 7: Snacking Poorly

Whether you shun snacks completely or choose foods that aren't healthy, you are not snacking wisely.

FOR THE NEXT THREE DAYS

Snack when you need to. While there's no point in snacking just on principle (and in fact, researchers know that snacks consumed when you're not hungry can make you gain weight), make a point of taking a break in midmorning and again in midafternoon. Ask yourself if you're hungry, and do a quick mood check. If you're feeling focused, that's fine. But if you're feeling even a little scattered or irritable, take that as an early warning sign that your blood sugar level has fallen too low. By the time you finish this book, you'll have literally hundreds of ideas for all kinds of satisfying snacks—sweet ones, creamy ones, salty or crunchy—but for now, start with some snack basics. Pack walnuts or almonds in snack-size Ziploc bags; stock your work fridge with drinkable yogurts or good-for-you snack bars, like KeriBars.

Diet Trap 8: "Loading up" at Lunch

Yes, you know that that enormous chicken wrap you ordered is more like three portions than one. (And why do they always put so much dressing on the "healthy" sandwiches, anyway?) But you're looking at an afternoon with back-to-back meetings, and you know that you won't have a minute to eat again until long after dark. You have to fortify yourself, otherwise you might keel over right there in the conference room.

FOR THE NEXT THREE DAYS

I call this "fearful eating." You have nothing to be afraid of—I swear you will not starve. Make a conscious choice to eat just until you feel you've had enough. Remember *slightly satisfied*? Again, listen to your HQ! And if you start to feel a little panicky—like "I may not get to eat again until 6:00 P.M.!"—remind yourself that you're prepared. Those almonds are right there in your pocket, remember?

Diet Trap 9: "Holding out" for Dinner

You may feel smug when you can say no to the usual 3:00 P.M. "Can I get you anything from Dunkin' Donuts?" rallying cry at your office. While sugary lattes aren't a great idea, neither is passing up a midafternoon snack because you can hang on until dinner. Of course, we know that you *can* hang on if you want to—you won't starve to death, and you can use your willpower to tough it out for a few hours. But look at the result. Instead of making what is considered a healthy choice at the restaurant, you're likely to pounce on the bowl of chips or bread basket the minute the waiter sets it on the table. So now you are overeating when your metabolism has slowed down from not eating all afternoon. A double whammy! You'll want to order an appetizer *and* a salad *and* an entree because, hey, you're hungry! And you were so good all afternoon. Or you rummage through the fridge and eat everything you can get your hands on—quickly. Even though your brain may be saying all the right things, your stomach is screaming like a three-year-old: "Feed me . . . now!"

FOR THE NEXT THREE DAYS

Give yourself a quick mood and HQ check a few hours before dinner. Don't feel hungry? That's fine—stop for a water break instead, and take a few deep breaths. Keep monitoring your mood and your appetite as dinnertime approaches. Even if dinner is less than an hour away, it's fine to have a healthy snack right now—again it's OK to ruin your appetite! I *want* you to ruin your appetite. Approaching dinner when your HQ is no greater than 6 will set you up for success, so you can make better choices.

THE THREE-DAY CLEANSE

If you feel you've already exorcised your dieting demons and are ready to plunge right in, you can spend your first three days on the Snack Factor Diet in a sort of "diet boot camp" instead. You can also try the hardcore three-day cleansing option *after* you've followed the steps above if you want to jump-start your weight loss; most of my clients lose about four pounds when they follow this. But this simple—and admittedly tough—diet will also help break the cycle of sugar and salt cravings, get you more used to letting your hunger guide your eating, and set you up for smooth sailing on the Snack Factor Diet. (And if you don't want to do this cleansing portion, I completely understand. I get a lot of weird looks when I mention the dandelion greens.) If you take a look and the three-day cleansing option is not something you want to consider, then skip ahead and begin the regular Snack Factor Diet starting on page 118.

UPON WAKING:
Large glass of water (10–12 ounces) with squeezed lemon

BREAKFAST:
3–5 egg whites (preferably boiled)
1 cup dandelion root tea (I like Traditional Medicinals teas, available at most big supermarkets and health food stores)

SNACK:
As many cucumbers and celery stalks as you want, but try to be conscious of what your HQ is
Large water with squeezed lemon

LUNCH:
Dark greens and lean meat or meat substitute, such as canned tuna or boiled chicken, sprinkled with 1 teaspoon ground flaxseeds or 1 teaspoon olive oil (you may add vinegar to your salad—balsamic and rice vinegars are both delicious)
Large water with squeezed lemon

SNACK:
Cucumbers, celery
Large water with squeezed lemon

DINNER:

Dark greens and lean meat or meat substitute, such as canned tuna or boiled chicken (again, you can add vinegar)

Large water with squeezed lemon

If you can find them—and they are usually sold at health food stores—eat dandelion greens as part of your greens for dinner or lunch. Researchers have found that wild greens are a richer source of nutrients like lutein and beta-carotene, and are wonderful for your health; some people believe they have greater cleansing power than other greens.

THE AT-A-GLANCE CHEAT SHEET

Now that you're three days in and armed with strategies to fight the most common problems in any diet—and are probably a few pounds lighter—you're ready to get a quick overview of what, specifically, you'll be doing for the next thirty days. Here's my part of the bargain: if you keep an open mind about snacking and follow my guidelines, I promise you'll lose weight. Really.

What's more, on this diet you're going to eat a delicious variety of foods that are healthy and satisfying, and—thanks to hundreds of tasty snacks I'll introduce you to later in the chapter—full of the best kind of nutrients. And you never have to sit staring at the clock, longing for your next meal or fantasizing about your favorite foods. (Some people actually dream about "forbidden" food when they are on an overly strict diet.)

Now, for your part of the bargain, follow these ground rules as best you can, and get your snack-friendly weight-loss program off to a flying start:

1. Eat breakfast every day, including a high-fiber starch and lean protein or healthy fat.

2. Include vegetables at lunch *and* dinner. Aim for dark greens at both meals. At dinner, aim for two vegetables—for example, mixed green salad and steamed broccoli. You need your veggies to add variety to your meal and to fill you up.

3. Always go for healthy fats. (See my list beginning on page 63.)

4. Always choose *lean* protein. (Turn to page 62 for great options!)

5. When eating breads, crackers, cereals, or chips, go for the highest fiber option. (See pages 54–55 for some terrific choices.)

6. Limit sugar and empty calories. Look for foods that offer the most nutrition possible, including fiber, vitamins, minerals, lean protein, and healthy fats.

7. Begin every day with water and lemon.

8. Stay hydrated throughout the day. Coffee and tea are fine, but make sure to hydrate with other fluids. Plain old water is ideal, but seltzer and herbal teas are good options, too. I also recommend one cup of green tea per day.

9. Aim for two calcium servings from the milk or yogurt choices I recommend.

10. Get some form of omega-3 fats every day, a fat found in flaxseed, walnuts, fish, and olive oil.

11. Always stay between 4 and 6 on your HQ. Eat slowly until just "satisfied."

12. Watch portion sizes. If you find yourself hungry at a meal, increase the vegetables and protein, but always stick to your portions of fat and starch.

13. Make "conscious indulgences" as instructed (more on conscious indulgences in Chapter 6).

14. Snack every day—need I say more?

15. Take every meal as an opportunity to eat well. Every meal is "Monday morning." Every meal is a time to start fresh. No matter where you are traveling or dining, or how busy you are, you are in control of almost every meal you eat. No excuses that there wasn't a healthy option. Look harder.

THE SNACK FACTOR DIET

Now that you've broken some bad habits, weaned yourself from sweets, gotten a good sense of your HQ and food timing, and accustomed yourself to eating both breakfast and snacks every day, it's time to buckle down and start the diet in earnest. You will see on the charts that follow what your daily portion allotments are, based on your weight category. After these guidelines, you will also see a sample daily plan to give you an idea of how the portions piece together to form a day of satisfying food.

You have several choices in how to structure your meals and snacks for the next thirty days:

1. You can piece together your own meals and snacks by choosing your portions of starch, milk/yogurt, lean proteins, vegetables, and fat from those listed in Chapter 4.
2. You can choose specific meals (pages 128–44) and snacks (pages 144–52) that fit into your chart perfectly. In this case, some of the thinking has been done for you.
3. If you are the type of person who wants to be told exactly what to do every day, then follow my thirty-day meal plan for your weight category, pages 152–54.

Putting It All Together

Let's pull out a new page of your food diary and start fresh, with a clean slate. This written format helps you plan your day and makes you keenly aware of addressing all four critical components of the Snack Factor Diet: portions, proportions, nutrient density, and HQ.

FACTOR THIS!

Although I give you the option of choosing meat substitutes such as soy, cheese, and legumes for your lean protein portion, I recommend sticking to the lean meats rather than substitutes as much as you can, especially during the first month. Although legumes and soy foods fit into an overall healthy diet and provide excellent nutrients, they are higher in calories and carbohydrates. For this reason, you want to be careful not to overdo them. If you are vegetarian, you will have to incorporate these foods daily. If not, I suggest limiting meat substitute–based meals to three times per week. Cheese is higher in bad fat, but also is a good source of protein and calcium. You can include cheese as part of your allotment of three weekly meat substitute–based meals.

If you weigh 150 pounds or less

- One serving of carbohydrates from the *starch* group
- Two servings of dairy from the *milk/yogurt* group
- Two or three 3- to 4-ounce servings of *lean protein* (NOTE: For meat substitutes you will choose 6 ounces from the legume list, 2 eggs or 6 whites, and 6 ounces from the soy list, except for edamame—you can choose 6 ounces.)
- 4 to 5 servings of *fat*
- Plenty of green *vegetables*, at least twice a day!

Here's what each day of your month on *The Snack Factor Diet* will look like:

MEAL	STARCH	VEGETABLES	MILK/ YOGURT	LEAN PROTEIN	FAT	FRUIT
BREAKFAST (Choose lean protein *or* fat at breakfast— not both)	✓		✓	✓	✓	
SNACK		✓			✓	
LUNCH		✓		✓	✓	
SNACK			✓		✓	
DINNER		✓		✓	✓	

For example:

MEAL	STARCH	VEGETABLES	MILK/ YOGURT	LEAN PROTEIN	FAT	FRUIT
BREAKFAST (Choose lean protein *or* fat at breakfast— not both)	4 oz. cooked oatmeal		8 oz. skim milk		1 tbsp. ground flaxseeds	
SNACK		jicama slices			1 tbsp. Keri's Lemon Dressing	
LUNCH Chef's salad		salad— romaine, cucumbers, asparagus, mushrooms		2 oz. lean ham 2 oz. turkey	1 oz. 50% reduced-fat Cabot Cheddar cheese	
SNACK			8 oz. FAGE Total 0% Fat Yogurt with cinnamon		10 almonds	
DINNER turkey burger		sliced onion and tomato salad, steamed spinach		4 oz. turkey burger	2 tsp. olive oil	

If you weigh between 151 and 180 pounds

- One serving of carbohydrates from the *starch* group
- Two servings of dairy from the *milk/yogurt* group
- Two or three 4- to 6-ounce servings of *lean protein* (NOTE: For meat substitutes you will choose 8 ounces from the legume list, 3 eggs or 9 whites, and 6–9 ounces from the soy list, except for edamame—you can choose 1 cup.)
- Four to 5 servings of *fat*
- Plenty of green *vegetables*, at least twice a day
- Fill up on vegetables and then increase your protein portion, based on your HQ

MEAL	STARCH	VEGETABLES	MILK/ YOGURT	LEAN PROTEIN	FAT	FRUIT
BREAKFAST (Choose lean protein *or* fat at breakfast— not both)	✓		✓	✓	✓	
SNACK		✓			✓	
LUNCH		✓		✓	✓	
SNACK			✓		✓	
DINNER		✓		✓	✓	

For example:

MEAL	STARCH	VEGETABLES	MILK/ YOGURT	LEAN PROTEIN	FAT	FRUIT
BREAKFAST (Choose lean protein *or* fat at breakfast— not both)	4 oz. cooked oatmeal		8 oz. skim milk		1 tbsp. ground flaxseeds	
SNACK		jicama slices			1 tbsp. Keri's Lemon Dressing	
LUNCH Chef's salad		salad— romaine, cucumbers, asparagus, mushrooms		3 oz. lean ham 3 oz. turkey	1 oz. 50% reduced-fat Cabot Cheddar cheese	
Snack			FAGE Total 0% Fat Yogurt with cinnamon		10 almonds	
DINNER turkey burger		sliced onion and tomato salad, steamed spinach		6 oz. turkey burger	2 tsp. olive oil	

If you weigh between 181 and 210 pounds

- Two servings of carbohydrates from the *starch* group
- Two servings of dairy from the *milk/yogurt* group
- Two or three 6- to 8-ounce servings of *lean protein* (NOTE: For meat substitutes you will choose 12 ounces from the legume list, 3 eggs and 3 whites from the egg list, and 8 to 12 ounces from the soy list, except for edamame—you can choose 12 ounces.)

- Four to five servings of *fat*
- Plenty of green *vegetables*, at least twice a day
- Fill up on vegetables and then increase your protein portion, based on your HQ

For example:

MEAL	STARCH	VEGETABLES	MILK/ YOGURT	LEAN PROTEIN	FAT	FRUIT
BREAKFAST (Choose lean protein *or* fat at breakfast—not both)	✓✓		✓	✓	✓	
SNACK		✓			✓	
LUNCH		✓		✓	✓	
SNACK			✓		✓	
DINNER		✓		✓	✓	

For example:

MEAL	STARCH	VEGETABLES	MILK/ YOGURT	LEAN PROTEIN	FAT	FRUIT
BREAKFAST (Choose lean protein *or* fat at breakfast — not both)	4 oz. cooked oatmeal 1 slice whole wheat toast		8 oz. skim milk		2 tsp. natural peanut butter	
SNACK		jicama slices			1 tbsp. Keri's Lemon Dressing	
LUNCH Chef's salad		salad— romaine, cucumbers, asparagus, mushrooms		2 oz. lean ham 3 oz. turkey 2 oz. roast beet	1 oz. 50% reduced-fat Cheddar cheese	
SNACK			8 oz. FAGE Total 0%Fat Yogurt with cinnamon		10 almonds	
DINNER turkey burger		sliced onion and tomato salad, steamed spinach		8 oz. turkey burger	2 tsp. olive oil	

And if you weigh more than 210 pounds

- Two servings of carbohydrates from the starch group
- Two servings of dairy from the *milk/yogurt* group
- Two or three 6- to 8-ounce servings of *lean protein* (NOTE: For meat substitutes you will choose 12 ounces from the legume list, 3 eggs and 3 whites from the egg list, and 8 to 12 ounces from the soy list, except for edamame—you can choose 12 ounces.)
- Five to six servings of *fat*

- Plenty of green *vegetables*, at least twice a day
- Fill up on vegetables and then, if you need to increase your protein portion based on your HQ, you can
- One additional snack from any category

MEAL	STARCH	VEGETABLES	MILK/ YOGURT	LEAN PROTEIN	FAT	FRUIT
BREAKFAST (Choose lean protein *or* fat at breakfast—not both)	✓✓		✓	✓	✓	
SNACK		✓			✓	
LUNCH		✓		✓	✓	
SNACK		✓			✓	
SNACK			✓		✓	
DINNER		✓		✓	✓	

For example:

MEAL	STARCH	VEGETABLES	MILK/ YOGURT	LEAN PROTEIN	FAT	FRUIT
BREAKFAST (Choose lean protein *or* fat at breakfast—not both)	8 oz. cooked oatmeal 1 slice whole wheat toast		8 oz. skim milk		2 tsp. natural peanut butter	
SNACK		jicama slices			1 tbsp. Keri's Lemon Dressing	
LUNCH chef's salad		salad— romaine, cucumbers, asparagus, mushrooms		2 oz. lean ham 3 oz. turkey 2 oz. roast beef	1 oz. 50% reduced-fat Cheddar cheese	

MEAL	STARCH	VEGETABLES	MILK/ YOGURT	LEAN PROTEIN	FAT	FRUIT
SNACK		celery sticks			2 tsp. natural peanut butter	
SNACK			8 oz. FAGE Total 0% Fat Yogurt with cinnamon		10 almonds	
DINNER turkey burger		sliced onion and tomato salad, steamed spinach		8 oz. turkey burger	2 tsp. olive oil	

FACTOR THIS!

WHY SO MUCH DAIRY?

Sometimes, clients are surprised when they see that I expect them to eat at least two servings of milk or yogurt every day. After all, they say, dairy products are a major source of not-so-great fats in most people's daily diets. That's true, but you'll notice that all my suggestions are very low in fat, and what you gain in calcium more than makes up for the health downside in small amounts of saturated fats.

And all of us need plenty of calcium. Throughout our teen years, when we're still actively storing it in our bones, we need about 1,300 milligrams each day, and between the ages of 19 and 50, we need at least 1,000 milligrams. If you're pregnant or lactating, you need 1,300 milligrams. If you're over fifty, you need 1,200 milligrams.

THE IMPORTANCE OF CALCIUM

There are plenty of obvious nutritional reasons why we need calcium. Calcium is the most abundant mineral in the body. It is essential for life. It is mostly stored in the bones and teeth, but is also found in blood and soft tissues (it helps to maintain blood pressure and enables muscle contractions including the heart). Calcium contributes to many vital processes, such as blood clotting and nerve transmission.

Calcium's role in helping us lose weight is unclear. Researchers from the University of Tennessee found that in a twenty-four-week trial, people who ate between three and four low-fat dairy servings per day lost significantly more weight than people who also cut calories but didn't eat dairy foods. But a study from the prestigious Mayo Clinic in 2005 found no evidence that a diet higher than 800 milligrams of calcium helped weight loss, beyond what would normally be seen by reducing calories.

But we do *know* that calcium protects bones. Osteoporosis causes 1.5 million hip fractures every year in the United States. And besides the 10 million Americans currently suffering from osteoporosis, 80 percent of them women, an additional 34 million have osteopenia, or low bone mass, which is often a precursor to osteoporosis. Getting enough calcium over a lifetime will help prevent bone loss and fractures. Consuming an adequate amount of calcium in the first two or three decades of life will help achieve maximum peak bone mass, which decreases the likelihood of osteoporosis later in life. In addition to the milk/yogurt sources of calcium listed earlier, there are plenty of nondairy sources of calcium:

Sources of Calcium	Milligrams
Kombu seaweed noodles (1 package)	860
Spinach, cooked (8 oz.)	245
Salmon, canned with bones (3 oz.)	181
Soybeans, boiled (8 oz.)	175
Tofu, extra-firm (3 oz.)	150
Navy beans, boiled (8 oz.)	128

Sources of Calcium	Milligrams
Almonds (8 oz.)	120
Oatmeal, cooked (6 oz.)	100
Sardines, canned with bones (3 oz.)	92
Kale, cooked (4 oz.)	90
White beans (2 oz.)	57
Cinnamon, ground (1 tsp.)	56
Figs, dried (2)	52
Orange (1)	52
Romaine (16 oz.)	40
Broccoli, cooked (4 oz.)	35

THOSE BETWEEN-SNACK MEALS!

For the next thirty days, if you are having trouble creating your own meals, choose from the following breakfast, lunch, and dinner options, and then choose two snacks from the hundreds of excellent and enticing choices listed later in the chapter. For the next thirty days one of your snacks should be a *Kick-start* snack (pages 145–46) and one should be a *Calcium* snack (pages 146–47). Feel free to replace a calcium snack with *any* snack you choose two times per week.

SNACK FACTOR MEALS

The following are examples of how your meals can be creative and simple at the same time and still fit into your Snack Factor Food Chart given earlier in the chapter. For example, the Cheesy Eggwich has a starch, milk/yogurt, and lean protein. Each part of the meal fits into your chart. Take a look!

These meals are meant to give you ideas. Also, they are easily duplicated in a restaurant or can simply be used as a guideline. For example, the Lite Cobb Salad can be ordered at any diner!

NOTE: The meals below are specific to the plan for 150 pounds or less. You can change the portions for your weight category. All meals serve one person. Finally, remember when a food is listed in a meal, refer to the portion lists in Chapter 4 for my favorite brands, or use any generic brand you love that fits the guidelines for calories and nutrients also given in Chapter 4.

Snack Factor Breakfasts

Cheesy Eggwich

> 1 large egg
> 1 light whole-grain English muffin (light whole grain has more
>   fiber and is heartier)
> ½ cup fat-free cottage cheese
> Black coffee or tea

HOW TO PREPARE

Place egg and 1 cup water in small saucepan and bring to a boil. Turn heat off and let sit 15 to 20 minutes.

Peel and slice the egg. Toast the English muffin. Spread cottage cheese on half of the muffin, add the egg slices, and top with other half.

Crunch 'n Cream

> ¾ cup Kashi Good Friends cereal
> ¾ cup plain nonfat yogurt
> 10 almonds, chopped
> Black coffee or tea

In a bowl, mix cereal, yogurt, and almonds.

Eggsadilla

3 egg whites, beaten with fork

1 La Tortilla Factory Low-Carb/Low-Fat original

1 oz. shredded light Monterey Jack cheese

1 tablespoon salsa of choice

Skim latte prepared with 8 ounces skim milk

Scramble the egg whites in a nonstick pan (sprayed with Spectrum or Mazola cooking spray) until cooked to liking. Place eggs on top of tortilla. Sprinkle with cheese and top with salsa. Roll up tortilla and enjoy.

FACTOR THIS!

I CAN HAVE EGG WHITES *AND* CHEESE AT BREAKFAST?
Yes! By doing this, you are technically having a lean protein *and* a fat, but because egg whites are so low in calories, you can choose a fat, too!

French Toast

1 slice whole wheat bread

2 egg whites, lightly beaten

Ground cinnamon

4 ounces Dannon Light & Fit Crave Control Yogurt

Black coffee or tea

Soak the bread in the egg whites. Cook in nonstick pan sprayed with Spectrum or Mazola cooking spray for approximately 1 minute.

Flip and cook on other side until lightly brown, another minute. Sprinkle with cinnamon and serve with yogurt.

Grilled Cheese with Tomato

1 (1-ounce) slice reduced-fat Cheddar cheese (or Swiss)

1 slice whole wheat bread

1 slice ripe tomato (see Note)

1 cup skim milk

NOTE: You may add vegetables to any breakfast.

HOW TO PREPARE

Lay the cheese and tomato on the bread. Place in toaster oven and toast until cheese melts.

Nutty Yogurt

5.3 ounces FAGE Total 0% Fat plain yogurt

7 walnut halves, chopped

3 tablespoons wheat germ

Black coffee or tea

HOW TO PREPARE

In a serving bowl, mix the yogurt, walnuts, and wheat germ.

Oatmeal Pancake

¼ cup egg whites (approximately 3 whites)

¼ cup old-fashioned or quick-cooking oats

½ cup fat-free cottage cheese

Pinch of ground cinnamon

HOW TO PREPARE

Beat the egg whites with a fork. Add the oats and cinnamon and blend well. Pour into a small nonstick pan (sprayed with Spectrum or Mazola cooking spray) and cook until almost set, approximately 2½ minutes, then flip and cook for approximately 30 seconds. Top with cottage cheese and sprinkle with cinnamon.

Peanut Butter Waffle

1 Kashi GoLean waffle
2 teaspoons natural peanut butter
1 cup skim milk

HOW TO PREPARE

Toast the waffle according to package directions and spread with peanut butter.

Smoked Salmon Sandwich

½ cup fat-free cottage cheese
1 slice whole wheat bread, toasted
3 ounces sliced smoked salmon
1–2 lemon wedges
1 teaspoon drained capers
Black coffee or tea

HOW TO PREPARE

Spread the cottage cheese on the toast and top with the salmon. Squeeze lemon juice over top. Garnish with capers.

Supercharged Oatmeal

1 Quaker Instant Oatmeal
1 cup skim milk
2 tablespoons ground flaxseeds

HOW TO PREPARE

Combine oats and milk and follow cooking instructions. Add flaxseeds.

Western Omelet

3 egg whites

¼ cup mushrooms and red peppers, chopped

½ cup fat-free cottage cheese

Hot sauce, to taste

1 slice light whole wheat toast

Black coffee or tea

HOW TO PREPARE

Combine egg whites with mushrooms and red peppers. Add to a preheated nonstick pan (sprayed with Spectrum or Mazola cooking spray). Cook until eggs are set. Transfer omelet to serving plate, add cottage cheese to one half of omelet, and fold over the remaining half. Add hot sauce. Serve with toast.

Snack Factor Lunches

Chef's Salad

Romaine lettuce

1 cucumber, peeled and chopped

Sliced raw mushrooms

Steamed or canned asparagus, chopped

2 hard-cooked egg whites, sliced

2 ounces lean ham or roast beef

2 ounces turkey sliced

1 teaspoon drained capers

1 ounce reduced-fat Cheddar cheese, shredded

Dijon vinaigrette

Combine all ingredients in a bowl. Add dressing to taste and toss salad.

Chopped Salad with Tofu and Soy

6 ounces firm tofu

Chopped vegetables of choice: carrots, cucumbers, celery, green
    pepper, cooked asparagus, jicama, hearts of palm

1 tablespoon soy nuts

Brown rice vinegar and lemon juice

Cut the tofu into small pieces and place in salad bowl. Add the vegetables and soy nuts. Toss with vinegar and lemon juice.

Lite Cobb Salad

2 slices turkey bacon

Romaine lettuce, chopped

2 hard-cooked egg whites, chopped

2 slices avocado (¼ avocado), chopped

Sliced cucumbers, tomatoes, carrots

Balsamic vinegar, to taste

Lemon wedge

Cook the bacon in the microwave by placing strips on a doubled paper towel and cooking on high for 1 minute. Check and arrange bacon for uniform cooking and continue for another minute. (Or place bacon in a cold frying pan and cook over low heat; turn often, remove grease, and cook until desired crispness.) Place lettuce in salad bowl and crumble in the bacon. Add the remaining salad ingredients. Drizzle with vinegar and sprinkle with lemon. Toss.

Roasted Chicken Lettuce Wrap

1 tablespoon Dijon mustard
2 large romaine lettuce leaves
4 ounces cooked chicken breast, skin removed
1 ounce part-skim mozzarella cheese, shredded
1 cucumber, peeled and chopped
1 red and 1 yellow bell pepper, chopped

HOW TO PREPARE

Spread mustard on two lettuce leaves. Evenly distribute the chicken between the lettuce leaves. Sprinkle the cheese on the chopped vegetables and evenly distribute on top of the chicken. Roll up lettuce wraps.

Shrimp Salad

Mixed baby greens
4 to 6 shrimp, steamed and peeled
2 slices avocado (about ¼ avocado)
2 hearts of palm spears (canned in water), sliced
1 lemon
Sea salt

HOW TO PREPARE

In a serving bowl, toss greens with shrimp, avocado, and hearts of palm. Squeeze on lemon juice and season with salt.

Simple Grilled Chicken Salad

4 ounces grilled chicken breast, skin removed
Romaine lettuce
Sliced carrots, cucumber, red onion
1 ounce goat cheese
Raspberry vinegar, to taste

Cut the chicken into bite-size pieces. Toss with the lettuce, vegetables, and cheese. Add raspberry vinegar and toss again.

Soup and Salad

1 cup black bean soup
Mixed salad greens
Sliced celery, carrots, tomato, onion
1 tablespoon Keri's Lemon Dressing (page 103)

HOW TO PREPARE

Heat the soup according to directions. Combine greens with vegetables in a bowl. Toss with dressing.

Steak Salad

3 ounces grilled lean steak
Baby spinach
Cherry tomatoes, halved
Chopped red onions
1 tablespoon Keri's Lemon Dressing (page 103)

HOW TO PREPARE

Slice steak and add remaining ingredients. Toss with dressing.

Tomato Mozzarella Platter

Green beans
1 ripe tomato, sliced
3 GG Scandanavian Bran Crispbreads (see Note)
3 ounces part-skim mozzarella cheese
2 teaspoons olive oil

HOW TO PREPARE

Steam the green beans until al dente and place at side of plate. Place two tomato slices on each cracker. Divide the mozzarella among the crackers. Drizzle olive oil over crackers.

NOTE: Crackers given as a "freebie."

Tuna Salad

1 (6-ounce) can chunk light tuna packed in water

1 teaspoon drained capers

Chopped celery, carrots

2 lemon wedges

1 ounce reduced-fat feta, crumbled

Romaine lettuce to taste

Balsamic vinegar

HOW TO PREPARE

Drain the water from the tuna. Place in a medium bowl with the capers, celery, and carrots.

Squeeze the lemon over and mix. Place mixture on a bed of lettuce and top with feta cheese. Sprinkle with balsamic vinegar.

Turkey Celery Rolls

1 ounce goat cheese

4 (4-inch) celery stalks

4 ounces sliced turkey (approximately 4 slices)

Crudite of carrots, red and yellow bell peppers

HOW TO PREPARE

Spread the goat cheese evenly on the celery sticks. Wrap the turkey slices around the celery. Garnish plate with crudité.

Crackers and Vegetable Spread

Romaine lettuce, 4 leaves

7 walnut halves

Chopped celery, carrots, yellow bell peppers, and radishes

1 cup nonfat cottage cheese

Pepper

2 GG Scandinavian Bran Crispbreads

HOW TO PREPARE

Line a plate with romaine lettuce. Smash the walnuts. Mix veggies and walnuts with cottage cheese, and add pepper to taste. Dollop cottage cheese mixture onto lettuce. Serve crackers on the side.

Snack Factor Dinners

Broiled Scallops

4 ounces sea scallops

Lemon pepper seasoning

Mixed green salad with sliced mushrooms, carrots, cucumber, and
    a dressing of 2 teaspoons olive oil, lemon juice, and sea salt

HOW TO PREPARE

Line baking pan with foil. Spray with Spectrum or Mazola cooking spray. Add scallops. Spray top of scallops with more cooking spray and sprinkle with lemon pepper seasoning. Broil 3 to 5 minutes or until cooked.

Broiled Salmon

4 ounces fresh or frozen salmon

1–2 tablepsoons Dijon mustard

2 tablespoons light soy sauce

Mixed greens with 1 tablespoon chopped walnuts and 2 teaspoons
of Dijon Vinaigrette (page 103)

Steamed spinach

Salt and pepper, to taste

HOW TO PREPARE

Preheat broiler. Spread the top of the salmon with mustard and
sprinkle with soy sauce. Place in a baking pan (sprayed with Spectrum or Mazola cooking spray) and broil for 8 to 10 minutes, or until
cooked through.

Broiled Tilapia

4 ounces tilapia or other white fish fillet

Sea salt

Pepper

1 lemon wedge

Paprika

Steamed asparagus

Mixed salad greens and a dressing of 2 teaspoons olive oil and
balsamic vinegar

HOW TO PREPARE

Preheat the broiler. Season the fish with sea salt, pepper, lemon
juice, and paprika . Broil 4 to 6 inches from the heat for 8 to 12 minutes, until done. If you prefer to bake fish, bake at 375°F to 475°F
for 10 to 12 minutes, depending upon thickness.

Chicken Parmesan

1 medium boneless and skinless chicken breast

1/2 cup marinara sauce

3 tablespoons grated Parmesan cheese

Steamed broccoli

Mixed greens with balsamic vinegar

Preheat the oven to 350°F. Spray chicken with Spectrum or Mazola cooking spray. Grill chicken 3 to 5 minutes per side until just done. Cover with sauce and sprinkle with cheese. Bake until the sauce is heated through.

Grilled Chicken Sausages

2 Han's All Natural Chicken Sausages
Steamed broccoli
Baby spinach salad with 1 ounce goat cheese or feta cheese with
drizzled fig vinegar

Cook sausages according to package directions.

Lemon Grilled Chicken

1 medium boneless and skinless chicken breast
1 tablespoon fresh lemon juice
1 teaspoon drained capers
1 teaspoon chopped fresh parsley (optional)
Steamed green beans

Place a nonstick skillet (sprayed with Spectrum or Mazola cooking spray) on medium-high heat. Add the chicken and brown on both sides, about 4 minutes per side. Transfer the chicken to a plate. Add the lemon juice and capers to the pan, swirl around to heat, and pour over the chicken. Top with parsley.

Pan-Roasted Filet of Beef

4 ounces lean filet of beef
Salt and pepper

Steamed broccoli

Mixed salad greens with 1 tablespoon Keri's Lemon Dressing
  (page 103)

HOW TO PREPARE

Preheat the oven to 400°F. Season the filet with salt and pepper to taste. Lightly spray an ovenproof nonstick skillet with olive oil spray and heat over medium-high heat until nearly smoking. Add the filet, cook each side for 5 minutes. Transfer the pan to the oven and roast 8 minutes more for medium rare. Let filet rest at room temperature while steaming the broccoli and tossing the salad with dressing.

Roast Pork Tenderloin

6 ounces pork tenderloin (see Note)

Salt and pepper

Steamed string beans

1 tablespoon chopped almonds

Fresh spinach and grated carrots with 1 tablespoon raspberry
  vinegar and 1 garlic clove, chopped

HOW TO PREPARE

Preheat oven to 450°F. Season the pork with salt and pepper to taste. Heat a large nonstick ovenproof skillet over medium-high heat. Add the pork and sear until all sides are brown, turning occasionally, about 5 to 7 mintues. Transfer the pan to the oven and roast until cooked through, about 15 minutes. Top the steamed string beans with the almonds and set aside. Toss the spinach and carrots with the raspberry vinegar and garlic, and season to taste. Slice the pork into medallions and serve with string beans and salad on the side.

NOTE: It may be easier to cook the whole tenderloin, in which case you can prepare it for two people, or eat half and refrigerate the other half for dinner or lunch another day.

Grilled Shrimp Kebabs

4 to 6 large shrimp, raw
2 teaspoons olive oil
¼ teaspon garlic salt
½ teaspoon pepper
Steamed asparagus
Mixed greens and 1 teaspoon Dijon Vinaigrette (page 103)

HOW TO PREPARE

Thread shrimp on skewers and lightly brush with the olive oil. Season with the salt and pepper. Broil 3 to 5 minutes per side, turning once.

Turkey Burger

4 ounces ground turkey
1 tablespoon chopped onion
1 egg white
¼ teaspoon garlic powder
¼ teaspoon salt
½ teaspoon pepper

HOW TO PREPARE

Mix all ingredients together and form a patty. Lightly coat a preheated skillet with Mazola or Spectrum cooking spray. Cook the burger for approximately 5 minutes on each side, making sure it is cooked through.

Turkey Taco Salad

½ onion, chopped
4 ounces ground turkey
1 teaspoon ground cumin
1 teaspoon chili powder
Pinch of ground cinnamon
Salt
Romaine lettuce, cleaned and chopped
2 lime wedges
2 tablespoons jarred salsa or pico de gallo
2 tablespoons plain fat-free yogurt

HOW TO PREPARE

Lightly spray a nonstick skillet with Mazola or Spectrum cooking spray. Preheat a pan and sauté the onion until translucent, about 3 minutes. Add the turkey, cumin, chili powder, and cinnamon. Season to taste wtih salt. Cook, stirring constantly, until the turkey is browned, 4 to 5 minutes. Place the lettuce on a plate and add the cooked turkey. Garnish with the lime wedges, salsa, and yogurt.

Veggie Burger

2 veggie burgers
1 medium zucchini, sliced lengthwise
Salt
Fig vinegar (or other flavored vinegar)
Mixed salad greens with 1 ounce goat cheese

HOW TO PREPARE

Preheat the oven and bake the veggie burgers according to package directions. Sprinkle the zucchini lightly with salt. Grill in a grill pan over medium-high heat until cooked through, about 3 minutes per side. Sprinkle the fig vinegar over the zucchini and serve with veggie burger.

SNACKS

Ah, the key to the Snack Factor Diet is the snacks! My whole food philosophy rests on the belief that snacks *anchor* your diet. The right nutrient-dense snacks, eaten at the right times, will keep your metabolism revved and will lead you to make wise food choices at all times. I'm done repeating myself; on to the quick ground rules and the many delicious options. But first, here's a Good Snacking Guide:

At-a-Glance Cheat Sheet

- During the first month you may choose one Kick-start snack and one Calcium snack every day. These snacks fit perfectly into your Snack Factor food chart. For example, a Kick-start snack is composed of a vegetable and a fat. You can also substitute *any* snack for your Calcium snack up to two times per week during the first month.

- You may be a breakfast-snack-snack-lunch-dinner person or breakfast-snack-lunch-snack-dinner or breakfast-lunch-snack-dinner-snack person. It doesn't matter so much as long as you *listen to your HQ* and eat consistently through-out the day. Much will depend on your work schedule, your life, and so on. And it may change from day to day.

- All snacks (aside from Kick-start snacks, which are meant to get you into the routine of snacking) will have at least 4 grams of fiber or 7 grams of protein or 5 grams of healthy fat; they are approximately 120 to 160 calories—just enough calories and nutrient density to keep your metabolism up and your tummy satisfied.

Kick-start Snacks

All of these snacks have slightly fewer calories and always include a vegetable (to fill you up) and a fat (to keep you satisfied). I recommend that you use these for one of your daily snacks during the first four weeks of your diet to kick-start your weight loss.

- *Asparagus spears:* Canned or fresh asparagus sprinkled with 2 teaspoons olive oil and sea salt.
- *Caprese snack:* Large tomato slice with a thin slice of fresh mozzarella and a fresh basil leaf.
- *Celery peanut butter crunch:* Celery sticks smeared with 2 teaspoons natural peanut butter.
- *Creamy celery crunch:* Two celery sticks, each filled with 1 wedge of Laughing Cow Light Garlic and Herb Cheese.
- *Crudités:* Sliced celery, cucumbers, and green peppers with 1 tablespoon Italian dressing.
- *Cucumber salad:* Cucumber slices tossed with 2 teaspoons olive oil, lemon juice, and rice vinegar to taste.
- *Cucumber salsa:* One cucumber peeled and sliced with ¼ avocado (cut into pieces) and 2 tablespoons lemon juice; salt to taste.
- *Jicama salad:* Sliced carrots and jicama mixed with brown rice vinegar, 1 teaspoon Dijon mustard, and 2 teaspoons olive oil.
- *Mexican dip:* Red and yellow bell peppers to dip in avocado salsa (¼ avocado mixed with 2 tablespoons jarred salsa).
- *Antipasto:* Roasted red peppers, artichoke hearts canned in water, with up to 12 olives.
- *Mini chopped salad:* Chopped celery, carrots, and cucumber sprinkled with lemon juice, 2 teaspoons olive oil, and sea salt to taste.

- *Seaweed wrap:* Sliced red and green cabbage with 1 table-spoon ginger dressing, rolled in a nori sheet.
- *Sweet slaw:* Shredded carrots and green cabbage tossed with 1 tablespoon slivered almonds and rice vinegar.

ON-THE-GO KICK-START SNACKS

On-the-go snacks are snacks that are easily purchased at most delis or grocery stores and come packaged and por-tioned for you. Or you can easily throw them in a snack-size Ziploc bag in your purse.

- Baby carrots and 10 almonds
- Earthbound Farm Organic Carrot Dippers
- Cherry tomatoes and one string cheese stick
- V8 juice and celery sticks

Calcium Snacks

- *Shake and nuts:* Dannon Light & Fit Shake with 10 almonds.
- *Latte*: Skim latte (8 ounces) sprinkled with cinnamon and 12 mixed nuts on side.
- *Cinnamon cottage cheese:* Mix ½ cup nonfat cottage cheese with 10 chopped almonds and ground cinnamon.
- *Coffee yogurt:* Mix 1 container plain nonfat yogurt with 1 teaspoon ground coffee.
- *Spicy cheese dip:* ½ cup whipped cottage cheese mixed with 1 tablespoon chopped nuts, ¼ teaspoon white horseradish; season with pepper to taste. Feel free to dip with celery sticks!
- *Flax cottage cheese:* ½ cup Light & Lively Cottage Cheese with 1 tablespoon ground flaxseed.
- *Peanut butter yogurt:* 1 (6-ounce) cup plain nonfat yogurt with 2 teaspoons natural peanut butter mixed in.
- *Fruit shake:* Dannon Light & Fit Shake mixed with 1 table-spoon protein powder and ½ cup ice; blended for a shake.

- *Soy shake:* 1 cup Silk Enhance soy milk with 2 teaspoons almond butter (or peanut butter) and ½ cup ice cubes blended.
- *Greek dip:* 1 6-ounce cup plain nonfat yogurt with ¼ cup peeled and sliced cucumber, ¼ sliced chopped avocado (also use 1 minced garlic clove if you like).
- *Chocolate pudding:* 1 (6-ounce) cup plain nonfat yogurt mixed with 1 Sugar-Free Swiss Miss chocolate packet and 1 tablespoon flaxseeds.
- *Yogurt and almonds*: FAGE Total 0% Fat yogurt with almonds.

ON-THE-GO CALCIUM SNACKS

Dannon Light & Fit Smoothie (1) and 10 almonds
Individual Light & Lively Cottage Cheese (1) and
   1 tablespoon chopped walnuts
Dannon Crave Control (1) and 10 almonds

SALTY SNACKS

- *Natural nachos:* Whole wheat tortillas such as those made by La Tortilla Factory, cut into quarters, sprinkled with sea salt, and baked for 10 minutes at 350°. Use an avocado salsa.
- *Turkey lettuce wrap:* Two ounces smoked turkey slices topped with 1 teaspoon chopped olives and rolled up in 1 romaine lettuce leaf.
- *Cheese and crackers:* Two fiber crackers spread with 1 teaspoon mustard and topped with 1 slice reduced-fat Swiss cheese.
- *Pizzettes:* Top 2 fiber crackers each with 1 tablespoon marinara sauce and sprinkle with grated Parmesan cheese. Microwave for 15 seconds.

- *Mediterranean mix:* Eight chopped olives, 1 tablespoon chopped walnuts, 4 cherry tomatoes, ½ teaspoon capers, and ½ cup chopped celery spread on endive leaves.
- *Smoked fish dip:* Cucumber slices dipped in 2 ounces smoked trout or whitefish and mixed with ½ cup plain nonfat yogurt.
- *Prosciutto wraps:* Two- to 3-ounce portion of prosciutto wrapped around cooked asparagus spears.
- *Turkey bacon:* Two or three slices, cooked.
- *Chicken sausage:* One- to 2-ounce portion of chicken sausage.
- *Chicken noodle soup:* Eight-ounce bag of tofu Shirataki noodles mixed with ½ cup chicken broth.
- *Caper spread:* ½ cup nonfat cottage cheese mixed with 1 teaspoon capers, ¼ cup chopped celery, and ¼ cup chopped carrots and spread on 2 fiber crackers.
- *Shrimp cocktail:* Four steamed shrimp in 1 tablespoon cocktail sauce.
- *Edamame:* 1 cup steamed or boiled edamame, with sea salt and pepper.
- *Endive boat:* Endive filled with 1 tablespoon whipped cottage cheese and 1 smoked salmon slice.
- *Cheese spread crunch:* Two Laughing Cow Light cheese wedges spread on GG Scandinavian Bran Crispbreads.
- *Artichoke hearts:* 4 canned artichoke bottoms, packed in water, sprinkled with 1 tablespoon Parmesan cheese.
- *Hearts of palm wrap:* ½ cup chopped hearts of palm wrapped with 2 ounces prosciutto slices.
- *Greek salad:* 1 cup chopped romaine, ¼ cup chopped tomato, and ⅛ cup chopped onion with 1 ounce reduced-fat feta cheese.
- *Mediterranean tomato:* 1 large tomato slice with 1 ounce crumbled goat cheese, drizzled with fig vinegar.

- *Turkey meatballs:* Two golfball-size turkey meatballs.
- *Honey ham:* Two or three slices lean ham with 1 teaspoon honey mustard.
- *Hummus dip:* Three tablespoons hummus with celery and carrot sticks.
- *Sardine salad:* One 3.75-ounce can King Oscar sardines on a bed of lettuce.
- *Tuna light:* One 3-ounce can chunk light tuna, packed in water, drained and mixed with lemon juice and pepper.
- *Whole wheat pita with hummus:* Half a small whole wheat pita, toasted, with 2 tablespoons hummus.
- *Tuna sushi:* 1 tuna hand roll with avocado, no rice.
- *Popcorn Parmesan:* Jolly Time 100-Calorie Pack Popcorn, sprinkled with 2 tablespoons Parmesan cheese.

ON-THE-GO SALTY SNACKS

SnackMasters Turkey Jerky (2 oz.)

Mountain America salmon jerky (2 oz.)

OhBoy Oberto beef jerky (1 oz.)

Tamari almonds (20)

Glenny's soy chips, Salt and Pepper flavor or BBQ flavor (1.3 oz.)

Roasted pumpkin seeds (1 tablespoon)

Sun-dried Tomato Basil Gardenburger (1 patty)

Peanuts in shell (15)

SWEET SNACKS

- *S'mores:* 1 tablespoon chocolate soy nut butter on GG Scandinavian Brand Crispbread topped with 2 mini marshmallows.
- *Banana peanut "ice cream":* ½ cup frozen pureed banana topped with 20 chopped peanuts.

- *Sweet 'n spicy "apple pie":* Small baked apple prepared with cinnamon and 1 tablespoon chopped walnuts.
- *Raspberry parfait:* 1 cup plain nonfat yogurt with 1 cup raspberries and 1 teaspoon vanilla extract.
- *Sweet potato fries:* Half a sweet potato cut into ⅛-inch strips. Place on baking pan sprayed with olive oil cooking spray. Sprinkle with cinnamon. Bake at 350°F. for 10 to 12 minutes.
- *Apples 'n dip:* One ounce nonfat ricotta cheese mixed with cinnamon and spread on 3 thin apple slices.
- *Creamy Figs:* Mix ½ cup nonfat cottage cheese with 2 (chopped) dried figs and dash of vanilla extract.
- *Berries and cream:* Mix 1 cup blackberries or raspberries with 6 ounces nonfat plain yogurt.
- *Roasted pear with topping:* Top ½ roasted pear with 6 ounces plain nonfat yogurt and 1 tablespoon chopped almonds.
- *Grilled grapefruit:* Section ½ grapefruit and sprinkle with 1 tablespoon chopped walnuts and ½ teaspoon cinnamon; broil for 1 minute.
- *Banana split:* Top GG Scandinavian Bran Crispbread with ½ sliced banana, sprinkle of cinnamon, and 2 ounces plain nonfat yogurt.

ON-THE-GO SWEET SNACKS
Vitalicious Chocolate Brownie (1) with 4 ounces skim milk
Glenny's Soy Chips, Caramel (1 bag)
Strawberry Chocolate Chip KeriBar (1)
Dannon Lite & Fit Shake and a small apple

Power Snacks

These snacks have a little more protein and carbohydrate, so they are good choices when you need an extra boost.

- *Trail mix:* Mix 8 chopped walnuts and 2 chopped dried apricots.
- *Wired-up wrap:* Mix 1 teaspoon almond butter with 1 teaspoon ground flaxseed and roll up in a small high-fiber tortilla.
- *Power-packed English muffin:* Spread ½ light whole-grain English muffin with 1 teaspoon natural peanut butter and ¼ cup low-fat cottage cheese.
- *Simply soy:* Sprinkle 1 cup edamame beans with sea salt.
- *Yogurt plus:* Mix one 5.3-ounce container FAGE Total 0% Fat yogurt with 2 tablespoons wheat germ.
- *Almond butter sandwich:* Spread 1 slice light whole wheat toast with 2 teaspoons almond butter.
- *Hard-boiled eggs:* 2, sprinkled with sea salt, and crudité.
- *Roasted chicken:* 3 ounces, no skin, dipped in mustard.
- *Deviled egg:* 1 hard-boiled egg yolk mixed with 2 tablespoons yogurt, fresh chives, and lemon juice. Spoon into halved whites and sprinkle with paprika.
- *Peanut butter mash:* Mix ¼ cup All-Bran cereal with 2 teaspoons natural peanut butter and ¼ cup skim milk, and microwave until mushy.
- *Baked chicken:* 1 frozen prebaked chicken breast, thawed and grilled.

ON-THE-GO POWER SNACK
KeriBar (1)

SMOOTH AND CREAMY SNACKS
- *Apple yogurt:* Mix 1 cup nonfat plain yogurt with ¼ cup chopped apple and 1 teaspoon cinnamon.
- *Chocolate shake:* Blend 1 cup skim milk with 1 tablespoon low-sugar chocolate (or vanilla protein powder) with 1 cup ice cubes.

- *Mexican pizza:* Spread 1 Laughing Cow Light Cheese wedge on 2 fiber crackers with a dollop of salsa on top.
- *Mediterranean dip:* Dip 1 cup red and yellow pepper slices in 2 tablespoons hummus.
- *Goat cheese sandwich:* Spread 1 ounce herbed goat cheese on 1 toasted light whole wheat slice.
- *Black bean dip:* Dip celery sticks in black bean puree.
- *Caper dip:* Mix ½ cup nonfat cottage cheese with 1 teaspoon capers and ¼ cup chopped celery.
- *Pacific roasted red pepper soup:* Add 1 tablespoon Parmesan cheese to individual soup.

ON-THE-GO SMOOTH AND CREAMY POWER SNACKS

Dannon Light & Fit Smoothie (1, and one 1-ounce string cheese)

FAGE yogurt with ¼ cup All-Bran cereal

Free Snacks

Whenever you feel you need an extra snack to keep your HQ between a 4 and a 6, you can help yourself to the following:

Crudités with Wishbone Salad Spritzer (10 sprays!)

Cucumber salad: 1 cucumber, sliced and peeled, and tossed with 2 tablespoons chopped red onion and rice vinegar

2 GG Scandinavian bran crispbreads (once per day)

A MONTH OF MENUS

If you're the type of person who doesn't want to have to think about what you're going to eat or prepare, look at the month of menus that follows. Recipes for the meals and snacks listed are found on pages 129–52.

	SUNDAY	MONDAY	TUESDAY	WEDNESDAY	THURSDAY	FRIDAY	SATURDAY
WEEK 1							
	B: Super-charged Oatmeal	B: Crunch 'n Cream	B: Eggsadilla	B: Peanut Butter Waffle	B: Western Omelet	B: Smoked Salmon Sandwich	B: Oatmeal Pancake
	S: Cucumber Salad	S: Mexican Dip	S: Crudités	S: Asparagus Spears	S: Celery Peanut Butter Crunch	S: Mini Chopped Salad	S: Caprese Snack
	L: Steak Salad	L: Lite Cobb Salad	L: Shrimp Salad	L: Soup and Salad	L: Chef's Salad	L: Turkey Celery Roll	L: Roasted Chicken Lettuce Wrap
	S: Cinnamon Cottage Cheese	S: Peanut Butter Yogurt	S: Shake and Nuts	S: Chocolate Pudding	S: Cottage Cheese and Walnuts	S: Latte and Nuts	S: Creamy Spinach Dip
	D: Turkey Burger	D: Broiled Tilapia	D: Filet of Pan-Roasted Beef	D: Chicken Parmesan	D: Grilled Chicken Sausages	D: Veggie Burger	D: Broiled Scallops
WEEK 2							
	B: Peanut Butter Muffin	B: Nutty Yogurt	B: French Toast	B: Cheesy Eggwich	B: Super-charged Oatmeal	B: Grilled Cheese with Tomato	B: Smoked Salmon Sandwich
	S: Carrots and Dip	S: Crudités	S: Celery Peanut Butter Crunch	S: Cucumber Salsa	S: Celery Peanut Butter Crunch	S: Cherry Tomatoes and Cheese Stick	S: Asparagus Spears
	L: Simple Grilled Chicken Salad	L: Vegetable Spread on Crackers	L: Turkey "Unsandwich"	L: Salad with Chopped Tofu and Soy	L: Simple Grilled Chicken Salad	L: Tuna Salad and Nuts	L: Tomato Mozzarella Platter
	S: Yogurt and Almonds	S: Latte and Nuts	S: KeriBar	S: Cinnamon Cottage Cheese	S: Yogurt and Almonds	S: Shake and Nuts	S: Natural Nachos
	D: Veggie Burger with Goat Cheese	D: Broiled Tilapia	D: Lemon Grilled Chicken	D: Turkey Taco Salad	D: Roast Pork Tenderloin	D: Broiled Scallops	D: Broiled Salmon

Key: B = breakfast   S = snack   L = lunch   D = dinner

SUNDAY	MONDAY	TUESDAY	WEDNESDAY	THURSDAY	FRIDAY	SATURDAY
WEEK 3						
B: Peanut Butter Waffle	B: French Toast	B: Eggsadilla	B: Crunch 'n Cream	B: Nutty Yogurt	B: Western Omelet	B: Oat-meal Pancake
S: Sweet Slaw	S: Seaweed Wrap	S: Crudités	S: Cherry Tomatoes and Cheese Stick	S: Sweet Slaw	S: Jicama Salad	S: Cucum-ber Salad
L: Lite Cobb Salad	L: Tuna Salad	L: Vegetable Spread on Crackers	L: Shrimp Salad	L: Steak Salad	L: Chef's Salad	L: Salad with Chopped Tofu and Soy
S: Fruit Shake	S: Shake and Nuts	S: Chocolate Pudding	S: Glenny's Soy Chips	S: Cinnamon Cottage Cheese	S: Flax Cottage Cheese	S: Choco-late Pudding
D: Grilled Chicken Sausages	D: Turkey Burger	D: Pan-Roasted Filet of Beef	D: Shrimp Kebabs	D: Chicken Parmesan	D: Turkey Taco Salad	D: Roast Pork Tenderloin
WEEK 4						
B: Peanut Butter Muffin	B: Grilled Cheese with Tomato	B: Nutty Yogurt	B: French Toast	B: Eggsadilla	B: Crunch n' Cream	B: Cheesy Eggwich
S: Seaweed Wrap	S: Sweet Slaw	S: Cherry Tomatoes and Cheese Stick	S: Cucumber Salsa	S: Caprese Snack	S: Cucumber Salad	S: Mini Chopped Salad
L: Roasted Chicken Lettuce Wrap	L: Steak Salad	L: Simple Grilled Chicken Salad	L: Lite Cobb Salad	L: Salad with Chopped Tofu and Soy	L: Soup and Salad	L: Tomato Mozzarella Platter
S: Soy Shake	S: Yogurt and Almonds	S: Chocolate Pudding	S: KeriBar	S: Flax Cottage Cheese	S: Coffee Yogurt	S: Jolly Time Popcorn and Parmesan Cheese
D: Lemon Grilled Chicken	D: Broiled Scallops	D: Broiled Salmon	D: Turkey Taco Salad	D: Grilled Chicken Sausages	D: Turkey Burger	D: Roast Pork Tenderloin

Key: B = breakfast   S = snack   L = lunch   D = dinner

BEYOND THE FIRST MONTH

After the first month on the Snack Factor Diet, you will add the following:

If you are losing weight but want or need to continue to lose then:

- Add one fruit portion per day (for example, add blueberries to your morning oatmeal)
- Add in one starch portion up to three times per week (for example, add ½ cup of whole wheat pasta to your dinner)
- Substitute your calcium snack up to three times per week for any snack and continue with your Kick-start Snacks for one of your daily snacks

If you feel great about your weight loss and would like to maintain it:

- Add on fruit portion daily (berries are always a great choice)
- Add one starch portion up to three times per week (for example, add a slice of multigrain bread to your lunch)
- Choose any of your snacks from the snacks listed (you are no longer limited to Kick-start Snacks for one of your daily choices), but keep in mind the benefits of calcium

If you are not losing weight as quickly as you would like:

- Continue on your first month plan for another two weeks
- See Chapter 7 for a refresher

Conscious Indulgences

Eating Out, Drinking Up,
and Sweet Splurges

Now that you have finished reading about all the delicious snacks and meals you can have as part of the Snack Factor Diet, I'm going to let you in on a little secret: I've designed the diet so that once or twice a week you get to indulge in a food that isn't normally part of the eating plan.

Why? Because everyone—even a weight-loss saint—gets a little bored now and again. And we should be able to enjoy indulgent foods. It's hard to feel as if you're constantly saying no to foods you've been saying yes to for years. The behavioral science behind this is straightforward. When people feel deprived or constrained, they tend to crave whatever is forbidden; that's why so many former Atkins dieters wound up diving face first into a baked potato, and why so many low-fat dieters fell off the wagon with a bacon cheeseburger. Forbidden fruit is a story that's as old as Adam and Eve: we always want what we can't have.

So I've outsmarted that ancient story. You can have practically anything on the Snack Factor Diet. I call these "conscious indulgences," and no matter what your forbidden fruit is, as long as you plan for it and have a calorically controlled portion, it will be fine. In fact, most people can have these little splurges up to twice a week and still lose weight, especially after the first month on the Snack Factor Diet. (Try to be as strict as you can with yourself for the first month because that will help eliminate your cravings for your old bad-habit foods and give you a chance to develop a real taste for the healthier alternatives.) But knowing that these indulgences are free for the taking when you need them makes you feel more powerful with every passing day.

Remember, this is *your* Snack Factor Diet, not mine. You're not avoiding that apple pie because you *have* to or because I told you to; you're avoiding it because you *choose* to. And if you were to have that slice of pie—maybe because you're at a favorite diner with an old friend or it's the thing Aunt Lulu always bakes when you come to visit—you won't have to feel as if you've gone off your diet. That makes it easier for you to take a small slice, savor it, and not feel as if you've done something naughty. And you will be *far* less likely to fall into the trap of black-and-white eating. And we all know what that feels like: "I've been good all week, and now I'm ruining it all with this piece of pie. I might as well take the biggest piece I see, and have ice cream on top."

It's also important to pay attention to the types of conscious indulgences you like best. For some of my clients, it's all about alcohol: they'll almost always use their indulgences to have a glass of wine or a cold beer on a hot day. For others, it may be something very sweet and decadent.

SIMPLE TRICKS TO HELP YOU ENJOY DINING OUT

Let's start with restaurants, since Americans are dining out (or taking out) more and more often. The average American goes to a restaurant 3.2 times per week, according to *Zagat*, with people in Los Angeles eating at restaurants the most (3.8 restaurant visits per week) and those in Philadelphia among the least (2.6). And for many people, eating in restaurants almost always means *over*eating. How can it not, with the jumbo portions so many restaurants serve these days? But you can stick with the Snack Factor Diet and still dine out with your friends, family, and business colleagues. The last thing I want to do is disrupt a routine you enjoy.

Dining out is easy if you choose wisely. You can eat out happily and feel great when you:

- Look for high-fiber starch options such as wild rice or whole wheat bread.
- Choose leaner sources of protein such as cod, pork tenderloin, or grilled chicken without the skin.
- Substitute heart-healthy monounsaturated fats, such as olive oil for saturated fats like butter.
- Order dressings and sauces on the side.
- Fill up on vegetables, preferably steamed.
- Go easy on alcohol and soft drinks . . . try substituting with other refreshing beverages, such as tea or seltzer.

And you can take the Snack Factor Diet anywhere by breaking each meal down to its core components and tracking it in your food diary.

Curious to see how that might work? At an American restaurant, for example, let's say you order a hamburger:

VEGETABLE: lettuce, tomato (in burger), and side salad

PROTEIN: beef, tuna, turkey, chicken, veggie, or bison

FAT: cheese (on burger) or dressing on salad

WITH STARCH: small baked potato or ½ bun (if you can, order a
sweet potato and whole wheat bun)

Or a grilled chicken Caesar salad:

VEGETABLE: romaine lettuce

PROTEIN: chicken

FAT: Parmesan cheese

WITH STARCH: breadsticks or ½ whole-grain roll (remember to
say no to croutons!)

Or a Cobb salad:

VEGETABLE: greens, cucumber, tomato, and side order of steamed
broccoli

PROTEIN: egg whites/grilled chicken

FAT: blue cheese (ask for it on the side) or avocado (or you can
have both, but just take half a portion of each)

WITH STARCH: whole wheat roll

FACTOR THIS!

SNACK FACTOR ON THE ROAD

The beauty of the Snack Factor Diet is that even when you're not at
home with your perfectly stocked pantry, if you rely on the four critical
components—portions, proportions, nutrient density, and HQ—you can
have a meal that fits into your Snack Factor food chart. For example, on
your next jaunt to Paris, rather than giving up and thinking you can't stay
on track—and beginning each morning with a chocolate croissant—

(continues)

you can have a Snack Factor breakfast. Opt for a piece of a baguette, a soft-boiled egg, and a café au lait. The baguette may not be whole wheat, but that's okay. Live a little!

This approach applies to foods from any kind of cuisine. But before we get to each kind of ethnic restaurant and some good choices in each, here are some dining-out tips to help you enjoy your lifestyle without jeopardizing your waistline!

BEFORE YOU EAT

- Never go to a restaurant with an HQ close to 10 (starving!). You have already slowed your metabolism, and chances are you will make poor choices for your main course (as well as eat the entire bread basket). Have a small snack beforehand, so you walk into the restaurant with your HQ around 6, tops.

- Never skip meals knowing you are going out for a nice dinner or to your favorite restaurant. This almost guarantees overeating and slowing your metabolism!

- Always drink a large glass of water before you get to a restaurant or as soon as you arrive. This will fill you up slightly and make you feel healthy.

ONCE YOU SIT DOWN

- Order foods that are baked, boiled, steamed, poached, roasted, or grilled. Stay away from fried and sautéed. Believe it or not, foods that are poached may be poached in fat! The same goes for boiled foods. Don't be afraid to ask what the food is poached or boiled in.

- Be patient! Don't dig into the bread basket. Instead, concentrate on your company. Feel free to ask the waiter to remove the bread or chips.

- Foods that are breaded, crispy, creamed, batter-dipped, or buttered are high in fat and high in calories. Make another choice! Other words to be aware of are *flaky, puffed, crispy, au gratin,* and *escalloped.*

- Beware of thick, rich sauces like hollandaise and béarnaise, or gravies. You'll learn to enjoy the real flavors of the foods you are eating if you eat them a little "cleaner"!

- The majority of places you go out to eat at will serve portions that are at least two times what they should be. Either split with someone or cut in half *immediately,* and tell yourself that eating the second half is not an option. Take that part home if you like. If you are very hungry, eat more of your vegetables, then protein, not another serving of bread or other starch.

- Fill up on vegetables and salads. They are high in vitamins and minerals. And the fiber content will help keep you full longer. It is easy to cancel out the positive attributes of vegetables by frying them or piling on fattening dressing. Try to order steamed.

- If you order salad, ask for the dressing on the side, and stay away from creamy dressings. Then, use 1 tablespoon dressing. (See portions chart, Chapter 4.) Plain balsamic vinegar or red wine vinegar tastes good, too! Try it with a little lemon and avoid the salad dressing calories altogether. Remember: vinegar is a freebie. Oil-based dressings like Italian and balsamic vinaigrette are often better choices than nonfat dressings. Nonfat dressings are often high in sugar and calories and not as satisfying. If you are eating a healthy meal, the good fat in a salad dressing is a healthier option.

- Go for soup! Soups are great as a filler, and many soups, such as vegetable or bean, are high in nutrients. Stay away from cream-based soups and choose broth-based ones instead.

- Remove fat from meat and skin from poultry. A 3-ounce chicken breast with skin has 167 calories and 6.6 grams of fat; without skin, it has 140 calories and 3 grams of fat. Need I say more?

- If you are really craving dessert, go for sorbet, mixed berries, or skim cappuccino; the best option is herbal tea. Think about how good you feel after eating a nice healthy meal, and stay strong. But if you must order dessert, make it a healthy one. Or use one of your "conscious indulgences" for the week and enjoy!

AFTER YOU'VE EATEN

- Try to digest your food before going to bed. Going to bed on a full stomach often makes you extra hungry in the morning. Plus, your body does not digest food as well if you go to sleep immediately following a meal.

- Walk home from the restaurant or around your neighborhood. A refreshing walk is a good way to help burn a few extra calories, but the real benefit may be how good it can be for your mind.

DINING OUT ON ETHNIC FOOD: BON APPÉTIT *AND* MANGIA!

Whether it's Italian food (which is officially America's favorite restaurant cuisine, according to a recent *Zagat* poll), the always-popular Chinese takeout, or elegant French fare, you can use *The Snack Factor* food planner to safely navigate any menu.

Italian Food
- Order an appetizer of fresh vegetables.
- Chicken and fish are lower in fat than most other protein sources.
- Choose a tomato-based sauce rather than a cream-based sauce.
- Choose vegetables as toppings for pizza, for pasta dishes, or as side orders.
- Order pizza with a thin crust instead of thick crust.
- Look for items that are lower in fat, including minestrone soup, or foods called "primavera," "cacciatore."
- Avoid high-fat items like lasagna, manicotti, or anything called "Alfredo" or "parmigiana."

Here are some sample Italian menus to use as a guide:

Chicken Paillard

VEGETABLE: Mixed green salad and steamed spinach
PROTEIN: Chicken, with a little marinara sauce
FAT: Olive oil (added to steamed spinach or mixed green salad)
WITH STARCH: Small side order of pasta

Mussels Marinara

VEGETABLE: Steamed broccoli, mixed green salad, and marinara sauce

PROTEIN: Mussels

FAT: Parmesan cheese on salad

WITH STARCH: Small piece of bread (of course, whole wheat if available)

Grilled Salmon

VEGETABLE: Steamed string beans, tomato and mozzarella salad

PROTEIN: Salmon

FAT: Mozzarella

WITH STARCH: Roasted potatoes

Chinese Food

- Start with a savory, clear soup. Nearly all soups on the menu will be delicious and low in fat.
- Select dishes that include vegetables or are entirely vegetarian.
- When ordering a dish that includes protein and vegetables, ask for more vegetables and less protein.
- If sharing dishes, order one vegetarian dish, such as steamed vegetables.
- Look for items that are lower in fat, including steamed brown rice (if you're having a starch), steamed chicken, or seafood or tofu with vegetables, steamed Chinese broccoli, green beans, spinach, watercress, or snow pea shoots/ stems with ginger, garlic, and mushrooms.
- Avoid fried items, which are very high in fat, and also steer clear of egg rolls, spare ribs, sweet and sour dishes, and egg foo young.

Some sample Chinese menus:

Steamed Broccoli or Mixed Vegetables and
Chicken/Tofu/Shrimp

VEGETABLE: Broccoli or vegetables
PROTEIN: Chicken/tofu/shrimp
FAT: Black bean or garlic sauce on the side
WITH STARCH: Brown rice

Chicken Lettuce Wrap and Pine Nuts

VEGETABLE: Lettuce and side of steamed mixed veggies
PROTEIN: Chicken
FAT: Pine nuts and sauce (ask for sauce on the side)
WITH STARCH: Brown rice (ask for no crunchy noodles with this dish!)

Mexican Food

- Avoid excessive amounts of cheese. Remove cheese toppings or ask for it on the side.
- Ask for sauces and dressings on the side.
- Order food with only one high-fat topping: cheese, guacamole, or sour cream.
- Substitute bean soup or stewed beans for refried beans (remember, beans are a protein substitute).
- Instead of a deep-fried dessert, order a Mexican coffee.
- Look for items that are lower in fat, such as soft flour tortillas, gazpacho, bean soup or bean chili, and salsa.
- Avoid items that can be very high in fat: tortilla chips, crisp taco shells, fried tortilla shells, nachos, refried beans, beef or cheese chimichangas, tacos, quesadillas, or tostados; also sour cream and flan.

Some sample menus:

Fajita

VEGETABLE: Peppers, onions, tomatoes, and salsa
PROTEIN: Chicken, shrimp, or beef
FAT: Guacamole or cheese
WITH STARCH: Flour tortilla

(Rice and) Beans and Veggies

VEGETABLE: Lettuce, tomato, and salsa, plus side of veggies, such
as squash, peppers, onions
PROTEIN : Black or pinto beans
FAT: Guacamole
WITH STARCH: Rice

Burrito

VEGETABLE: Lettuce, tomato, and salsa
PROTEIN : Chicken, shrimp, beef, or beans
FAT: Guacamole or cheese
WITH STARCH: Tortilla (ask for no rice and no beans, unless
beans are your protein substitute in burrito)

French Food
- Avoid cream soups.
- Fill up on salads and vegetables.
- Ask for the salad dressing on the side.
- Remove the visible fat from red meat and skin from poultry.
- Look for items that are lower in fat, including bouil-
labaisse, coq au vin, salad Niçoise, ratatouille, or grilled
fish.

- Avoid items that can be high in fat: French onion soup, duck, foie gras, quiche, and fondue. Also stay away from entrees served with hollandaise, béarnaise, and béchamel sauces, beurre blanc, and anything described as "au gratin."

Some sample menus:

Bouillabaisse

VEGETABLE: Mixed green salad
PROTEIN : Fish
FAT: Dressing on salad
WITH STARCH: ½ small roll

Coq au Vin

VEGETABLE: Ratatouille and side order of steamed haricot verts
PROTEIN : Chicken (no skin!)
FAT: Wine sauce in coq au vin (best to ask for on the side and add 1 tablespoon!)
STARCH: Small baked potato

Deli Food
- Choose Dijon or deli mustard instead of mayonnaise.
- Most sandwiches can feed at least two people; share a sandwich, or eat half a sandwich and save the other half for another meal, or order extra slices of bread and make two or three sandwiches (for other people) with the filling.
- Add lettuce and tomato or other vegetables from the salad bar, such as sprouts, grated carrots, sweet peppers, pickles.
- Look for items lower in fat, including turkey breast, ham, or roast beef sandwiches on whole wheat or whole wheat

pita bread; grilled chicken; vinegar-based coleslaw; and bean salads made with vinaigrette.

- Avoid items that can be very high in fat: tuna, chicken, or egg salads; coleslaw, potato, and macaroni salads; chicken wings and ribs.

Some sample menus:

Grilled Chicken

VEGETABLE: Steamed mixed vegetables

PROTEIN : Chicken

FAT: If veggies and chicken seem "clean," then add 2 teaspoons olive oil or sprinkle Parmesan cheese on your veggies

STARCH: 1 slice wheat bread

Open-faced Turkey Sandwich or Turkey-Topped Salad

VEGETABLE: Garden salad

PROTEIN : Turkey

FAT: Avocado or cheese on sandwich or dressing on salad

STARCH: 1 slice whole wheat bread

Japanese Food

- Start with miso soup or another clear, savory soup and a seaweed or green salad.
- Choose leaner proteins, such as the less fatty cuts of tuna.
- Avoid tempura dishes and anything else deep-fried.
- Look for items lower in fat, including sushi, sashimi, seaweed salad, and steamed rice.
- Avoid items that can be very high in fat: tempura, deep-fried vegetables, or sushi that contains deep-fried items or cream cheese.

Some sample Japanese menus:

Spicy Tuna Roll

VEGETABLE: Green salad

PROTEIN: Tuna in roll and side of edamame, and 2 to 4 pieces sashimi

FAT: Spicy sauce in roll or dressing

WITH STARCH: Rice in roll

NO STARCH: Order roll with no rice, and ask that it be wrapped in cucumber; or skip roll and increase sashimi to 6 to 8 pieces

California Roll

VEGETABLE: Side of seaweed salad or green salad

PROTEIN: Crab in roll and 2 to 4 pieces sashimi or chicken yakitori appetizer

FAT: Oil in seaweed salad or dressing and avocado in roll

WITH STARCH: Rice in roll

NO STARCH: Order roll with no rice, and ask that it be wrapped in cucumber; or skip roll and increase sashimi to 6 to 8 pieces

Tofu Salad with Carrots and Hijiki

VEGETABLE: Carrots, Hijiki

PROTEIN: Tofu

FAT: Dressing

WITH STARCH: Shu mai (4 pieces)

Indian Food
- Indian cuisine contains a multitude of lean, savory dishes with a great variety of seasonings.
- Avoid creamy sauces and cheese-laden dishes.

- While most Indian restaurants offer plenty of vegetarian and vegan choices, these can be deceptively high in fat; ask the waiter how these vegetable dishes are prepared.
- Try the flavorful chutneys and yogurt dressings.
- For dessert, try some flavorful Indian tea.
- Look for items lower in fat, including grilled lean meats, steamed basmati rice, tandoori chicken or fish, tikka, vindaloo, and dal (lentil) dishes such as dal makhani; chana (chickpea) masala; dosas (light crepes made of rice and lentils; oven-baked breads (naan), and raita (diced cucumber and tomatoes in spiced yogurt).
- Avoid items that can be high in fat: creamy sauces, coconut milk sauces, deep-fried samosas (meat, potatoes, and vegetables wrapped in pastry); fried bananas; saag paneer (spinach and cheese), and fried breads, such as poori.

Some sample menus:

Shrimp or Chicken Tandoori

VEGETABLE: Steamed spinach

PROTEIN: Shrimp or chicken (request white meat only)

FAT: Yogurt dressing

STARCH: Pappadam bread, made with lentils and usually baked

Chicken or Fish Vindaloo

VEGETABLE: Raita (diced cucumber and tomato in spiced yogurt)

PROTEIN: Chicken or fish

FAT: Spiced yogurt

STARCH: Pappadam bread

Thai Food

- Avoid peanut sauce and coconut sauce; instead, request tamarind sauce.
- Order dishes prepared with basil, chile, or ginger.
- Avoid fried foods.
- Start with a salad.
- Look for items lower in fat, including basil rolls or Thai rolls (not fried); satay; steamed mussels; tom yum goong soup; green papaya salad; Thai beef salad; and yum yai salad.
- Avoid items that can be very high in fat: fried meats or tofu, fried noodle dishes, and anything made with coconut milk.

Sample menu:

Steamed Chicken, Shrimp, or Tofu with Mixed Vegetables

VEGETABLE: Mixed vegetables (broccoli, snow peas, carrots)
PROTEIN: Chicken
FAT: Black bean sauce
WITH STARCH: Rice

Fast Food

- Order a chicken sandwich or hamburger with no mayonnaise, dressing, or sauce.
- Remove the skin and fatty wing off rotisserie chicken; even though the chicken is not fried, some marinades are oil based and highly salted and full of sugar.
- Order a kid's meal.
- Order a side salad.
- Order skim milk or water.
- Ask for a list of nutritional information at the counter;

more and more chains, including McDonald's, are offering nutritional breakdowns of their menu items.

- Look for items that are lower in fat, including submarine sandwiches with lean meats and vegetables, grilled chicken sandwiches, small broiled hamburger, and salad.
- Avoid items that can be high in fat: cheeseburgers, hamburgers, sandwiches with sauce or mayonnaise, fried fish or chicken, baked potato with cheese, sour cream, or bacon bits, French fries or onion rings, shakes and soft drinks, and Danish pastries or pies.

Some sample menus:

Wendy's Chicken Caesar Salad

VEGETABLE: Lettuce
PROTEIN: Chicken
FAT: Parmesan cheese (skip the dressing)
STARCH: If you must, croutons

Subway Grilled Chicken and Baby Spinach Salad

VEGETABLE: Red onions, tomatoes, cucumber slices, green pepper strips, carrots
PROTEIN: Chicken
FAT: Olives (add vinegar to salad to dress)
STARCH: Small baked potato

McDonald's Asian Salad with Grilled Chicken

VEGETABLE: Asian salad mix
PROTEIN: Chicken
FAT: Newman's Own Light Balsamic Vinaigrette

HERE'S LOOKING AT YOU! CHEERS! YOU CAN ENJOY A DRINK!

As with eating in restaurants, drinking alcohol worries many people who are trying to lose weight. They're concerned that they'll have to swear off drinking for the duration. Maybe they're convinced that a glass of wine with dinner is an integral part of civilized living. Or maybe unwinding with their spouses over a cocktail each night is a long-standing and important ritual. Whatever the reason, don't worry—it is possible to work alcoholic beverages into the Snack Factor Diet and still successfully take off the weight.

It's just not realistic to think of alcohol as something that is permanently off-limits, but it does require a little strategic thinking. Here are my rules for imbibing:

1. Cut the nights of drinking in half. Make each drink count. It is very easy to order a drink every time you go out or crack open a bottle of wine every time you turn on the oven to begin cooking. Let's say you are going to a movie; maybe you could avoid that glass of wine with dinner. Save it for the next night when you are at your friend's cocktail party or are cooking a romantic dinner for your new love interest. If you plan your week and even make a mental note about when you will *really* want a drink, you should have no problem cutting the nights you choose to drink in half!

2. Cut the number of drinks you have in half each night you drink. Skip the first drink (you will end up eating less as well). Instead of having that predinner waiting-at-the-bar drink, order a seltzer with a squeeze of lime and save your drink calories for dinner.

3. Pay attention to the different calorie counts in drinks. Some are far more indulgent than others. (You can substitute

an alcoholic drink for your fruit serving if you choose the lower calorie alcoholic drinks.) You will be allowed three "conscious indulgences" a week once you have lost your weight. Alcohol is part of these indulgences. And as far as nutrient density goes, your best bet is red wine, which contains beneficial antioxidants.

Keri's Favorite Party Drinks

I love these because they let you enjoy that celebratory drink for close to 100 calories or less.

Drink	Serving Size	Calories
White wine spritzer	4 oz.	40
Seltzer with about 1 oz. vodka and squeeze of lime	11 oz.	64
Whiskey/Gin/Rum/Vodka (80 proof)	1.25 oz.	80
White wine (table)	4 oz.	96
Vodka (about 1 oz.) and diet tonic	11 oz.	102
Whiskey/gin/rum/vodka (100 proof)	1.25 oz.	102
Red wine (table)	4 oz.	103
Beer (light)	12 oz.	104

Don't see your favorites? Here's a list of some other popular drinks, with calorie counts so you can choose wisely.

Cocktail	Serving Size	Calories
Martini (gin, dry vermouth)	2 oz.	119
Bloody Mary (vodka, tomato juice, lemon juice, Worcestershire sauce, Tabasco sauce, lime)	4.6 oz.	120
Whiskey Sour (whiskey, lemon juice, powdered sugar, cherry, lemon slice)	3 oz.	125
Cosmopolitan (vodka, triple sec, lime juice, cranberry juice)	2.5 oz	132
Beer	12 oz.	144
Gin and Tonic (gin, tonic water, lime)	7 oz.	170
Port Wine	4 oz.	179
Chocolate Martini (vodka, crème de cacao)	2.5 oz.	188
Vermouth	4 oz.	188
Screwdriver (vodka, orange juice)	7 oz.	208
Mai Tai (dark rum, light rum, sweet and sour mix, grenadine, 151 proof rum, ice)	4.9 oz.	306
Piña colada (Malibu rum, pineapple juice, cream)	8 oz.	312
Eggnog	8 oz.	342
Rum and Coke (rum, cola)	12 oz.	369
Planter's Punch	8 oz.	397
Margarita (coarse salt, lime, white tequila, triple sec, lime juice, crushed ice)	6.3 oz.	407
Daiquiri	8 oz.	422
Mudslide (Vodka, coffee liqueur, Irish cream, vanilla ice cream)	12 oz.	820

Mixers	Serving Size	Calories
Tonic	4 oz.	40
Orange juice	4 oz.	55
Cranberry juice	4 oz.	73
Coca-Cola	8 oz.	96

AND FINALLY—WHAT'S FOR DESSERT?

For some people, giving up alcohol to lose weight is a piece of cake. For them, the biggest struggle is usually, well, giving up cake! For those of you with more than a few sweet teeth, you've probably been thinking about crème brûlée ever since I mentioned it back in Chapter 2. If that's the case, you can have it—just work it in as your conscious indulgence. But think hard about making that choice. A rich dessert like that is a biggie. At most restaurants, it packs about 550 calories. But if it just wouldn't feel like your birthday without it, go ahead and have a small portion of it.

But I'll make a prediction here. As you get more and more adept at eating the Snack Factor way, and more cunning about finding the best nutrient bargains out there, crème brûlée will lose a little of its appeal. Instead, I bet you'll be Googling for a low-fat version of the classic. (I've had great ones that come in at just 200 calories, making it a more reasonable indulgence.) And just as likely, you'll think "Tonight, my sweet tooth will be happy with the dish of berries." Or maybe you'll go home and have a mug of herbal tea or a nonfat yogurt with some chocolate sauce drizzled in.

What makes me so confident? Because, after years of working with so many clients, I've really come to understand the power of listening to your body. Once a person understands why he or she is craving the crème brûlée, for example—that it's not because the person is hungry but because he or she just loves the feel of something sweet and creamy in the mouth—the person will happily substitute fat-free ricotta blended with cocoa powder. Once you get that the reason you want a hot-fudge sundae (at around 750 calories) is to feel a little sinful, you'll discover you feel just as naughty when you choose a single Godiva chocolate truffle, at 149 calories.

That's why I call these "conscious indulgences." Yes, they are *indulgences*, and they let you kick up your heels a little so that you never feel like you're in dietary handcuffs. But they are also *conscious*, meaning they make you think a little about what you're craving and why. As long as you continue to lose weight on the Snack Factor Diet, *after* the first month *you can have three conscious indulgences per week.*

Little Splurges Mean a Lot

When it comes to giving yourself a treat, it's important that it both satisfies your specific craving and doesn't cause a diet disaster.

WHAT TO LOOK FOR

- Approximately 100 calories or less
- If it has fiber, it is always a better choice

KERI'S TIP

Choose an indulgence when you are truly craving the indulgence. Don't just say "Oh, I am allowed to eat this so I can eat it every night!" The point is to learn what a portion of your favorite craving (indulgence) is. Why no crème brûlée, cheesecake, or chocolate molten cake? Because just *one* bite would put you in the 100-calorie zone! If you absolutely must go for one of these highly decadent indulgences, take three very small bites and enjoy each one!

KERI'S PICK

Berries! OK, not always enough to satisfy the craving, but if you get used to berries being your indulgence at the end of your favorite meal, you will truly learn to steer clear of the high-fat, high-sugar options. A cup of berries and a soothing cup of tea can actually hit the spot if you give them a chance!

At-Home Indulgences

TYPE AND PORTION SIZE

Apple, baked, with cinnamon, chopped walnuts (1 tsp.), and honey (1 tsp.)

Raspberries (8 oz.) and nonfat yogurt (6 oz.)

Sorbet (4 oz.)

Strawberries (3) and chocolate soy nut butter (2 tsp.)

BRAND AND PORTION SIZE

Edy's Slow Churned Rich and Creamy Vanilla Ice Cream (4 oz.)

Health Valley Amaretto Style Low Fat Biscotti (2 cookies)

Health Valley Low Fat Healthy Chips Double Chocolate Chip Cookie (3 cookies)

Julie's Organic Sorbet Bars (1 bar)

No Pudge Fat Free Brownie Mix (one 2-inch brownie)

No Pudge Giant Sundae Cone (1 cone)

Skinny Cow Fat-Free Fudge Bar (1 bar)

Vitalicious VitaBrownie

Restaurant Indulgences

TYPE AND PORTION SIZE

Almond biscotti (1)

Fortune cookie (2)

Fruit and cheese (1 apple, sliced, and ½ oz. cheese)

Mixed berries (8 oz.) and zabaglione (2 oz.), or just mixed
   berries by themselves!

Skim cappuccino (6 oz.) with cinnamon

Yogurt (6 oz.) and honey (2 tsp.)

HOW TO HANDLE YOUR OTHER FAVORITE INDULGENCES

You'll be amazed how you can fit in just about anything
to your Snack Factor Diet. Pizza? Bagel and lox? Chips?
Here goes:

PIZZA

I have a lot of clients who say "I am loving the diet, but I
think I need pizza!" Think about the parts of your meal:

STARCH: Pizza dough (whole wheat is best). Is it a slice of whole
   wheat bread? No—but, you can substitute on occasion for
   your serving of starch.

PROTEIN: Cheese (You can pat off the excess oil with a paper towel)

FAT: The cheese is your meat substitute *and* your fat portion;
   chances are there is more than a meat substitute serving

VEGETABLE: Large green salad with mixed vegetables; use any
   vinegar as dressing. Add vegetables to your pizza.

NOTE: Make the pizza your "side." Have the salad be the main
dish on your plate. You will eat the pizza slower and you will fill up
on the greens.

BAGEL AND LOX

STARCH: 1/2 whole wheat bagel (Let's try to make it a real whole
   wheat bagel)

PROTEIN: 3 ounces lox

VEGETABLE: Feel free to add tomato, capers, and onion; squeeze
   some lemon on top!

FAT: No, because at breakfast you choose fat or meat

MILK/YOGURT: 4 ounces whipped cottage cheese on burger

CHIPS

Remember the guidelines for starchy snacks? Yes, of course, soy chips are the better option, but if you must have the fries or chips, aim for that 1-ounce portion and make the rest of your meal perfectly Snack Factor acceptable: 3-ounce lean filet of beef; 1 ounce potato wedges, fries, or chips; plus steamed spinach and mixed green salad with 1 tablespoon vinaigrette.

Troubleshooting

Common Triggers, Successful Controls

Within a day or two of starting the Snack Factor Diet, you'll probably start getting glimpses of what your particular weaknesses are—the exact size and shape of your dieting booby traps. Maybe recording your HQ is making you keenly aware of how often you eat when you're not even hungry, and you aren't sure why and what to do about it. Maybe you catch yourself feeling resentful about smaller-than-you're-used-to portions. Whatever obstacles you're facing, the most important advice I can give you is to not feel bad about it. *Of course*, you have dieting issues—that's why the weight crept up on you in the first place. So stop beating yourself up, right now.

I need to remind you—over and over—that you're not in this alone. All around you are people who have struggled to lose weight and then have succeeded. This chapter will help you pinpoint your personal stumbling blocks—the things that trigger you to overeat and the tricks that other people have found very helpful that can give you some control.

I need also to tell you that mastering these stubborn little food demons is the key to lasting success. Sometimes, I hold back a little here because I don't want to discourage people who are having initial success with the diet. You will lose weight following this program. But the sad truth is that unless you start to see these changes as a permanent overhaul to the way you eat, chances are you'll gain the weight back. In fact, 90 percent of people who diet and lose weight regain it—and then some.

That's why everything about the Snack Factor Diet, from the liberal timing of what you eat to the big array of foods and recipes, is geared to your eating at sustainable levels. If you wanted, you know you could go on an extreme diet and lose more weight in less time. But I'm betting you also know that that strategy is utterly pointless. Most people regain that quick-loss weight very soon. So this time, promise to make your eating changes *personal*. I had one client, for example, tell me that she normally ate out in restaurants four nights a week. Her plan for losing weight was to stay home for a month.

"No way!" I told her. "You shouldn't change your life so dramatically unless you plan to change it for the long haul." Instead, we came up with a compromise plan for her to stay home one more night per week on a regular basis. And on the nights she's home, she has gotten into the habit of preparing quick meals and not ordering in her old high-fat, high-sodium meals.

The most important thing to remember—and I can't say this to you often enough—is that if you are *patient* and *consistent*, you can lose the weight and keep it off forever. Let me repeat that: *patient* and *consistent*. There are times when a client will come in, discouraged. That's because it *is* hard to make all these changes, and sometimes the results don't come fast enough to make us feel it's worth it. But it is worth it!

"Remember, you may be on the verge of a two-pound weight loss," I'll tell them when they seem stuck. "Every time you eat a piece of cheesecake, you don't see the scale move up (thankfully). And it works the same way in reverse. Even though you feel like a hero because you said 'No, thanks' to every dessert that came your way this week, that doesn't mean you're going to get rewarded with a ten-pound weight loss. It just doesn't work that way. Just as we gain weight slowly, we lose it slowly."

So here are some of the most common *triggers* and questions—the things that make people feel so frustrated that they want to eat more than they should. For each one, I've provided a *control*—sometimes, it's what I call a food control, like substituting healthier soy chips for one of those days when you feel like you'd kill for a bag of potato chips. Other controls are nonfood, like recognizing when you're eating more because you're upset with someone. In fact, it's really helpful to make a list. I've started one, just to give you a sense of what I mean, but feel free to substitute control ideas that you think will work best for you.

FOOD CONTROLS
(FOR WHEN YOU MAY TRULY BE HUNGRY OR FOR WHEN YOU KNOW YOU HAVE TO PUT SOMETHING IN YOUR MOUTH)
Herbal tea
A cool glass of lemon water
Thin slices of vegetables, tossed with rice vinegar to make a slaw

NONFOOD CONTROLS
(FOR WHEN YOU RECOGNIZE—CONGRATS!—THAT YOU HAVE NO HUNGER [LOW HQ] BUT NORMALLY WOULD EAT)
Taking a catnap
Meditating for 5 minutes

Stepping away from the computer and walking around
the office
Calling a friend
Getting a 10-minute massage
Reading a magazine

If you don't see the problems that trouble you the most below, e-mail me at www.snackfactordiet.com, and I'll make sure I try to address it, either on my Web site or in my next book.

TRIGGERS

"I find myself eating even when I know I'm not hungry."

First you nibble some pretzels, then you eat an apple. Then you open and close the fridge six times. ("Is there any of that Chinese food left? Oh, look! I forgot we had ice cream!") Many dieters can relate to this kind of "picking" or midnight mischief.

Look at your food diary. Did you feel deprived all day, and is picking a way to satisfy some little craving—something salty maybe, or something sweet?—that you didn't address with the foods you chose? Is this emotional eating? Maybe you're worried about a problem at work or are trying to avoid thinking about a silly argument you had with your sister the other day. Just recognizing emotional eating is a huge step in the direction of learning to control it.

Whatever the reason for this kind of random eating, one of these five control techniques should work:

- **Imagine** the feeling of accomplishment if you don't eat the ice cream, versus the feeling of disappointment if you do eat it.

- **Visualize** yourself in your favorite pair of jeans or your new off-the-shoulder dress. Close your eyes and picture yourself, and think how great you'll feel when those clothes fit just right. Some clients even put up a picture of their favorite clothes, right there on the refrigerator.

- **Wait** five minutes. Just wait and be patient. Once you resist the initial temptation, you'll be amazed that it may have passed completely.

- **Think** about how long it would take to burn off the ice cream. You'd probably finish it in less than two minutes, but you'd have to run an extra three miles to make up for it.

- **Drink something.** Maybe a cup of herbal tea or a glass of lemon water will satisfy your desire to taste something soothing.

- **Do something.** Doing something good for you is much easier than *not* doing something. Often, the act of deprivation itself is more frustrating than actually not eating the item of food. So by doing something proactive for yourself, you negate that deprivation feeling. Sit down and indulge in some guilty-pleasure television, or better yet, do 10 minutes of situps. Sometimes, it's enough to inspire you to be healthy and stay on track.

"I'm not just picking—I'm always hungry at night."

If you're always hungry at night—if your HQ is a 7 or higher two hours after dinner or your last snack—the answer is simple. You need to consume more during the day. Did you eat your high-fiber starch with breakfast? How much protein are you eating at lunch? Try increasing lean protein at lunch and more veggies at dinner. Still not enough? Try adding a bit more protein to your evening meal, too.

"I get stuck in meetings (or in the car) and can't always eat lunch. Then, I am starving and binge!"

Many people—me included—can't always schedule work around our optimal eating patterns. And for lots of people, taking a regular lunch hour is just *never* going to happen. In fact, for some people in this situation, one solution is to give up on lunch altogether, and just build your day around a breakfast-snack-snack-snack-dinner plan.

Always, always, always have something with you that you can eat as a healthy, satisfying snack. When you're on the go, carry premeasured Ziploc bags with almonds or walnuts, turkey jerky, KeriBars, or a piece of fruit—an apple or a pear. At your office, if you've got access to a refrigerator, make sure you stock it with nonfat yogurts (many people think the drinkable ones make the perfect snack), cut-up vegetables with peanut butter or cottage cheese for dipping, and even hard-boiled eggs.

If you feel it's rude or inappropriate to snack during a business meeting, no matter how discreetly you can nibble on your nuts, don't be shy about excusing yourself. This happens to me all the time, and I've learned that it really is OK for me to keep my next appointment waiting for two minutes—which is about how long it takes to eat a snack, take a drink of water, and grab a deep breath or two. It's much more productive than letting myself get too hungry because I'm in a rush. We all have the right to take care of our health, and that two-minute snack break may prevent you from going totally overboard at your next meal.

"I go to a lot of cocktail parties and can't resist those pigs in blankets. Or anything fried, for that matter."

Cocktail parties do present many challenges, even if they can also be a lot of fun. For one thing, it's easy to feel kind of trapped, and when the waiters circulate with little hors d'oeuvres—pigs-in-a-blanket, tiny fried chicken legs, crispy wontons, or those rich little pastries stuffed with shrimp in cream sauce we nibble on one or two (or seven or eight) of these notoriously high-fat foods. Sometimes those foods are just too hard to resist.

Make sure your eating is on track all day, and have a snack before going, so that when you arrive at the party, your HQ is no more than 6. Then, assess the scene. As you're mingling, walk around the entire party. Look over the buffet table and each chafing dish. It's so easy to panic and think, "Holy guacamole! There's nothing here but chips and fried food!" But with so many people watching their weight these days, it's a very rare party where there isn't *something* healthy to snack on, and often there are beautifully elaborate selections of vegetables and other healthy alternatives. Check out what waiters are carrying as they circulate through the room. (You can even ask what else is waiting on trays back in the kitchen; promise he won't care if you ask.)

"I hate a lot of foods listed in this diet."

No problem. If these don't appeal to you, simply find replacement foods in each category that do. Remember, even with the guidelines of lean protein, high-fiber starches, fruits and vegetables, and heart-healthy fats, there are still hundreds, if not thousands, of good options. Follow the guidelines I've laid out for making the healthiest choices for each category of food and refine it to your tastes.

"I don't have a lot of time to prepare healthier snacks or meals. And besides, I don't really like to cook. "

You don't have to. The convenience craze has swept all across the supermarkets of America, even into the whole-foods aisle. There's no shame in eating many—if not all—of your snacks and meals from foods that are already prepared. I had one client who did just fine using almost nothing but foods that came frozen from the supermarket—vegetables, whole-grain waffles, Boca Burgers, even some frozen entrees. (I'm leery of most regular supermarket brands. Calorically, they're fine, but they tend to be full of preservatives and sodium.) She didn't even want to be bothered washing fresh fruit, so she used frozen berries! I'm an especially big fan of the Cascadian Farms frozen fruits and vegetables, which are organic. For some people, yogurt is just a substitute for a snack they didn't have time to prepare themselves; for others, opening that yogurt counts as cooking. As long as you're keeping your HQ between 4 and 6, getting the right amount of essential nutrients and losing weight, it's fine.

"But I *love* to cook. And I feel as if some of these recipes are a little too . . . simple."

Again, no sweat. Most of my recipes *are* simple. Remember, I've developed them for on-the-go people who say they just don't have time to fuss over what to prepare or who dine out often. Genuine foodies—you people who can actually taste the difference in grades of olive oil and know exactly when truffle season begins and ends—can still have fun cooking on the Snack Factor Diet. Look for recipes that are heavy on vegetables, include a little healthy fat, with as much spice or seasoning as you like. In terms of preparation, words like *grill*, *bake*, and *broil* are usually good signs that it's a healthy recipe. Once you've created your weekly masterpiece or two, measure it out into individual portions that follow the guidelines set out in Chapter 4. And when the other Snack Factor people are munching on boring old celery sticks and peanut butter, you can dig into your afternoon bouillabaisse.

"I love to eat . . . and eat . . . and hate to diet, but I want to lose weight."

Knowledge is power, and since you already know that for you, the key is being able to eat as much as you want of as many foods as possible. I'm sending you straight back to Chapter 3—focus on nutrient density. By focusing on foods you can eat plenty of, you'll limit that feeling of dieting. (I know, for some people, feeling as if they have to police themselves 24/7 is just a huge drag.) Your next mission is to head right to the nearest supermarket and spend a half hour in the produce aisle. Since vegetables are your only "unlimited" food, let your imagination run wild. Never tried kale? Buy some. Think bokchoy sounds tempting? Toss it in your cart. The zucchini looks good to you, as do the string beans? Experiment with vegetable stews. Vinegar-based slaws are also an excellent choice.

Some clients who fit this category tell me that for them, "kitchen sink" salads are really important. That's a salad that has so many different ingredients that it feels like a huge treat, not a penance. Think of all the little extras you can toss into a salad to make it not just satisfying but also amazing: sunflower seeds, capers (they taste like olives, with no fat), sliced radishes, bean sprouts, artichokes, bamboo shoots, jicama to add some crunch, scallions, turkey bacon bits, or beans. Adding a chopped spicy chicken sausage adds lean protein, and makes the meal feel like more of a splurge.

And lots of people who love to eat are most successful just by becoming masters of the *simple substitution*. Let's say you are the kind of person who just loves a bag of Fritos now and again. Well, once you discover how tasty some of the soy chips are (my favorites are made by a company called Glenny's), you may never need to eat a Frito for the rest of your life. I'm not kidding—that's how good they are! And lots of people have decided that a skim latte can give them the same thrill that they used to get from one of those supersugary frappucinos.

"I *still* think snacking will make me gain weight."

Ah, a stubborn one. If you've read this far, I bet you're willing to give me the benefit of the doubt. Will you try the Snack Factor Diet for one week? If you don't lose weight (which is extremely unlikely if you follow it as directed), you'll be right and I'll be wrong. But if you do lose, usually two to three pounds the first week, I'll be right—and you'll be on the road to a healthier you.

"How do I know if a food is nutrient dense?"

It depends on the type of food, but it helps me to remember to think in terms of threes. For starches and fruit, the best clue is fiber: look for foods that provide at least 3 grams per serving. While fiber itself has no nutrients, it slows down digestion. The energy contained in the food is then released more slowly into our bloodstream. For proteins, the best guide is how lean a food is: aim for foods with 3 grams or less of fat, such as chicken, turkey, shrimp, and egg whites. And for *fats*, whenever possible, look for those that offer omega-3s, such as flaxseed, walnuts, or fish or are sources of other healthy fats such as mono or polyunsaturated fats. (You can even buy eggs from chickens that have been fed special grains, so that each egg provides150 mg of omega-3!)

"Do I need to have a protein, fat, and carb at every meal and snack?"

Not at all—in fact, you'd probably make yourself loopy if you tried! Single-food snacks are often perfect for busy people: a hard-boiled egg, for example, or a handful of nuts or an apple. But wonderful things do happen when you combine them. Add 2 teaspoons of natural peanut butter—which is only 70 calories and rich in protein and fat—to those apple slices, and see how much more satisfying it feels. Mash the egg with spicy mustard and spread it on a fiber cracker. Or toss the nuts into a nonfat plain yogurt with some cinnamon. Single-food snacks aren't bad, but these complex snacks are better and will make you feel more satisfied, for a longer period.

"I can't figure out my HQ."

Lots of people struggle with this, especially in the beginning. It's because so many of us are used to eating when we're not hungry. I've had clients confess to me that the only way they can tell when they're hungry is that they start snapping at their coworkers, and that the only way they know when they're full is that they have to discreetly reach down and unbutton their jeans at the table!

That's why the numbered HQ scale is so helpful. *Everyone* can remember what a 1 feels like—that horrible "What-have-I-done, I'm-never-eating-again!" feeling. And most of us can pretty quickly recall a time when we reached 10, allowing ourselves to get so hungry that we felt absolutely frantic. (When that happens to little kids, they often just sit down and howl.)

Now close your eyes and imagine a 5—a completely neutral feeling. You're neither hungry nor full; in fact, at this precise moment, you could care less about food. For the first day, just think in terms of those three scores—1, 5, or 10. But the next time you go to eat something, stop for a second and ask yourself again: Do I feel slightly hungry? Very hungry? Extremely hungry? And after you've finished eating, ask the same questions: Do you feel satisfied? Or like you had a few bites too many?

Your goal—and for some people, it takes a few days—is to recognize when your HQ gets to 6: hungry enough that you feel you should eat something. It's time for a snack or meal. And as you're eating, your goal is to take it slowly enough that you're conscious of your hunger being satisfied. That way, when your HQ hits 4 ("I feel satisfied without a bit of fullness") you can put down your fork.

"I'm getting bored."

If you've been successfully losing weight for two weeks and you feel as if you're tired of the diet, I've got a few ideas.

First, go back and skim through the sample menus. Most of us read recipes the way we read menus in restaurants: we pounce on what appeals to us at the moment but ignore the rest of it. See if there are other ideas that tempt you. Ask yourself what, especially, you're craving. At about two weeks, for example, lots of clients have had it with the same salad, over and over. So I give them an assignment: experiment with some new ways to eat cooked vegetables, to boost your variety.

Second, maybe you're suffering from Goody Two-shoes syndrome. You've been eating like a saint and, frankly, your taste buds are telling you it's time to go to Vegas. Maybe you are eating too well and forgetting that you are supposed to have fat at lunch? That you can eat red meat?

In fact, the next time you find yourself bored, plan one of those little treats found in the conscious indulgence section of Chapter 6. Maybe you should promise yourself a bistro hamburger this weekend. Or have an ice cream with your kids. If you've been losing weight consistently, as long as these are rare events in your week, you should be fine. And often, knowing you've given yourself permission to have that burger makes it much easier to go for the grilled fish instead.

"I miss my 'comfort' foods."

It's great that you're aware of how you use food to soothe your emotional upsets. And all of us know how a certain food—chicken noodle soup, macaroni and cheese, meatloaf and gravy—all say, "There, there, it's going to be okay." In a perfect world, we'd all be so emotionally healthy that we wouldn't turn to food for comfort, any more than we'd turn to close friends for, let's say, vitamin D. But for most of us, at some point food does equal love. The first step is recognizing when it's happening. When you feel ready to start eating out of emotion instead of hunger, it often helps to replace food-love with real love. Call a friend or family member for a quick chat, and see if you still feel the need to fire up the pasta pot.

If you do, analyze what it is about your comfort food— the creaminess, the saltiness, the crunch?—and see if there's another more nutrient-dense solution, a simple substitution. Here's a healthier way, for example, to do grilled cheese: use two slices of light whole wheat bread, reduced-fat cheese, and nonstick spray, and prepare in a skillet. (You can also use a George Foreman grill.) If you'd like, add tomato slices to make the meal feel richer.

And if all that fails, by all means, make this comfort food a planned indulgence.

"I'm traveling, including a six-hour flight."

Travel is tough, for many reasons. Besides early check-in and long security lines, airports are notorious for having nothing but overpriced diet disaster zones. Fast food is everywhere, and while many offer salads, they're also loaded with full-fat cheese, sour cream, fat-laden croutons, or fattier meats. Most people spend up to three hours without food before they even get on the plane—no wonder there are so many reports of "airport rage!" And once you've fastened your seat-belt, if you get fed at all, chances are your meal will be full of bad fats, sodium, and other chemicals—and taste foul.

As with every other situation, all I can do is urge you to be gentle with yourself, and arm yourself with as much healthy food as you think you might need. Don't laugh, but I even suggest that my clients carry snacks aboard in those little insulated lunch bags. (OK, it's about as fashion forward as or-thopedic shoes, but it's easy to stash it in your carry-on.) Bring along two or three sets of snacks in case you're delayed. Try crackers and peanut butter, an apple with a slice of cheese, or a bag of soy chips. And don't forget your water! And remem-ber, if you can't bring food on the plane, make sure you eat a "real" meal as close to departure as possible and save the snacks you brought along in case you get stuck at your terminal.

I even suggest clients fill their luggage with plenty of those nonperishable snack foods: try buffalo jerky, trail mix (12 chopped pecans and 2 chopped dried apricots), oatmeal packets, tuna packets, KeriBars. It will help keep you closer to your routine while traveling.

"I always pick at what my kids eat."

Some parents really wrestle with this one. They hate to see food go to waste, and they really like the foods they serve their kids—the chicken fingers, the peanut butter and jelly, even the fishsticks. I highly recommend making your kids foods off limits! Make it law not to eat your kids' food.

If there is a lot of hanging around the kitchen while the kids eat, there is another solution. Prepare yourself something to eat so you can "pick" at your food while they're eating. An easy your-allowed-to-pick food is cucumber salad. Simply peel and slice cucumbers and add rice vinegar.

But there's a bigger philosophical question behind this trigger. Why are so many of us feeding kids food that we consider off limits ourselves? The answer is that it's easy: they're foods kids love, even if they're not the healthiest. And I'm certainly not saying you should put the whole family on the Snack Factor Diet—you'd have a rebellion. But as you get more practice with the healthy concepts behind the Snack Factor Diet, I bet you will be surprised at how often you will decide to give the same foods you're eating to the rest of the family—after all, they should be eating more vegetables, whole grains, and lean proteins, too. Then if you pick at your kids' food, who cares? It's the same meal you are preparing for yourself.

But until then, just tell yourself those foods are off limits.

"I'm starting to plateau."

Most people will lose between ten and twelve pounds in thirty days on the Snack Factor Diet—more if they've got more weight to lose and more if they haven't been on other diets recently. (That's because chronic dieting meddles with people's metabolism, and it can take a few weeks of following a healthy diet for it to get back to normal.) But it can be very frustrating, especially as you get closer and closer to your goal weight, to have weight loss slow to less than a pound a week.

The only thing I can do is urge you to remember that weight loss is a long-term process. This is not something you'll work on for a month, and then forget all about. You probably didn't gain the weight in a month-long period, so it's not realistic to expect to lose it that quickly. And—as tedious as it is—there's plenty of evidence that the more slowly you shed those extra pounds, the more likely they are to stay gone.

I've said it before, and I'll say it again: please be patient and consistent. If you do the right things often enough, the weight will come off, sooner or later.

"I'm not losing weight."

Not losing weight at all is different from losing weight too slowly. If you've been on the Snack Factor Diet for a week and haven't lost any weight, it's time to reassess. First, look back at your food journals, retracing your steps each day. One client, for example, kept forgetting to record the cappuccinos she ordered twice a day at work. Even though they were made with skim milk, they added 200 invisible calories per day— enough to prevent her from losing weight.

Next, double-check the portions of food you're eating. Another client of mine simply misread the portion size on peanut butter and was eating two *tablespoons* on her toast in the morning and on her celery in the afternoon, not two teaspoons. (That's another 200-calorie difference!) "You know," she said sheepishly when she realized her error, "I *thought* it was kinda hard to swallow." And finally, even if you've been eating nothing but big salads, ask yourself if they've gotten a little too big. Too much chicken thrown in? Overdoing the dressing? Even overeating the good stuff can interfere with weight loss.

"I was doing fine, and then the season changed, and I swear I'm eating more. And I'm not losing weight as fast. Is this my imagination?"

No! Researchers at the University of Massachusetts tracked nearly 600 men and women for a year, and found that most people do vary their diet and exercise habits by season, eating an average of 86 calories per day more in the fall than during the spring, when their calorie intake was lowest. Body weights fluctuated, too, and were highest during the winter, when—big surprise—physical activity was lowest. And an Israeli study confirmed that during the winter months people are more likely to consume animal fats, resulting in higher cholesterol levels.

One way to guard against those shifts, experts say, is to let seasonal changes naturally influence our diets. That means in spring we should eat as many of the tender, leafy green vegetables as we can. In summer we can take advantage of the plentiful fruits and vegetables, and in autumn we can add plenty of harvest foods—apples, squash, pumpkin, and onions. Not only does that strategy guarantee you're getting the fullest range of antioxidants and phytonutrients, but it also boosts your variety level. Seasonal variations are one more way to make sure you're not digging yourself into food ruts.

Here are a few other ways to protect yourself from seasonal triggers, including lots of socializing, more time with family, and the availability of so many tempting seasonal treats. Try some of these controls:

- **Schedule your workouts—in pen.** Don't let the social and shopping demands of the season disrupt your workout.

- **Plan your indulgences—then indulge.** If you're the kind of person who lives for Christmas cookies, that's fine. Know that you'll have some when the plate is passed around. But that doesn't mean you have to eat all the gooey pies and drink the eggnog, too.

- **Stagger your social stresses.** Between stuffy office parties and a little *too* much time with your family, it's easy to feel as if you're spending the whole month of December making small talk instead of doing what matters most to you. Don't forget to make time for the stuff you really love, whether it's an evening listening to a live chorale performance or an afternoon ice skating.

- **Double your commitment to your food diary.** In a study by the Center for Behavioral Medicine in Chicago, groups of overweight people were divided into two groups: some recorded their food intake and some didn't. Those who didn't write down what they ate gained weight over the weeks that included Thanksgiving, Christmas, and New Year's Day. Those who did keep a diary? They continued to lose weight right through the holidays!

"It's not the holidays that get me. I do worse in the summer."

I've frequently had clients tell me that summer presents more weight-loss challenges, and I think there are several reasons. While it's true that it's much easier to get out and be active during those easy, breezy summer months, so many of us are hung up by the way we look. While other people race to the beach or the pool, we're tortured by the idea of putting on a swimsuit, or even walking around in shorts. And the kind of parties we go to in the summer, as fun as they are, tend to be all-day eating marathons, whether it's your company picnic or your best friend's famous Fourth of July barbeque. Again, look back on the tips I gave about going to cocktail parties. The same strategies apply: don't go hungry—go at an HQ of 6. Scope out the scene when you arrive at a party, and decide which are the healthiest choices. And try to bring a healthy dish!

SOME FAQS (FREQUENTLY ASKED QUESTIONS)

"I am confused by good fat vs. bad fat."

You're not alone! Fat is such a confusing topic that some people say, "What's the use—I may as well eat lard!" But it can be this simple: avoid as many animal fats, like butter and fatty meats, as possible as well as processed fats, such as hydrogenated and trans fats, found in packaged foods.

Fatty fish, like salmon, tuna, and sardines, are an exception, and you should try to have at least one to two servings a week for those beneficial omega-3s, either in salmon or other fish, including sardines. You can also get these incredibly beneficial omega-3s in flaxseed and nuts.

Other good fats include monounsaturated fats that are labeled as heart-healthy—olive and canola oil are among the most common (and the tastiest). Experts believe that the worst fats of all are trans fats, which usually contain the word *hydrogenated* somewhere on the label. But since the FDA now requires all food made with trans fats to carry a warning label, those have gotten easier to avoid.

"What's the difference between good and bad carbs?"

The word *carbohydrate* covers such a wide range of foods that it still frustrates me when I hear people say they try to boycott carbs. Please note that a small apple—that's right, those things that keep the doctor away—has 15 grams of sugar! Cantaloupe, oatmeal, corn on the cob, nutty wholegrain breads are all carbs, and it seems a shame to write them off as if they were as empty as potato chips, pretzels, or doughnuts. So my best advice is to read labels. Shun foods made with white flour or too much sugar if they offer little in the way of fiber or nutrition. And make sure the carbs you do eat contain lots of fiber.

I wish I could say that eating this way is as easy as it sounds, but food marketers can be devious. By just throwing in a little whole wheat flour, for instance, they can write "whole wheat" in the ingredients. (My clients are sometimes horrified when they learn that the "wheat" bread they've been buying is just white bread with a little whole wheat flour and a lot of caramel coloring.) Look at the ingredient label. You want to look for "100 percent whole wheat" or another whole-grain like whole oats; then it is likely to be a whole-grain food.

And don't forget to check on fiber. Even foods that seem a

little high in sugar can be good choices if they are especially fiber rich. The point is that with all foods, zeroing in on one ingredient as either good or bad isn't all that helpful; when it comes to food and to labels, look at the big picture!

"I exercise a lot. Can I eat more?"

Probably. The Snack Factor Diet is calculated on how many servings you should have based on your current weight, and it assumes that most people are basically sedentary—the workout is a bonus. I've also worked closely with professional athletes, and I was a college athlete myself, so I know how intensely people sometimes train. And I want you to workout.

So if you're training extensively, experiment and always listen to your HQ. You may need to increase your serving of protein and vegetables, and maybe even add one more starch. Pay special attention to how you feel after your workout. You should feel appropriately fatigued, not completely spent. And if you feel spacey or have a hard time concentrating, that's a sign that you're underfed. Be certain that you're taking in extra fluids to compensate. For most people, eight to ten glasses a day is plenty. But if you just spent five and half hours pushing yourself on a 100-mile bike ride, you'll need much more.

Using these guidelines, reassess after a week goes by. If you've lost at least two pounds, you know you're at the right level. If you haven't, cut out that extra starch serving each day, and see how you do in weight loss the following week.

I've also got a special word for superexercisers—people who like to believe they can always eat what they want because they can "out exercise" any extra calories they consume. In theory, that's fine. But the reality is that many clients come to me quite fit but still struggling to lose weight. In those cases, it's important to work on changing food behaviors, not just adding more miles on the treadmill or extra sessions at the gym. For example, a client of mine is really fit and works out at least an hour a day, six days a week. But he's also likely to have at least two glasses of scotch when he gets home from work. Not surprisingly, he's stuck. As hard as he's exercising, he is just spinning his wheels as far as his weight loss goes until he eliminates the source of the extra calories.

As long as you're exercising most days of the week, I'm not asking you to change your training schedule. But I am asking you—particularly if you exercise six days a week or more—to focus on weight loss through diet, not by increased workout time. More than that, you're at risk for overtraining, and as with other diet quick fixes, you'll only put the weight back on when you go back to "normal." Our goal is to fix the food habits that stand between us and our dream weight, not to outsmart them with more time at the gym.

"How do I incorporate alcohol?"

You can enjoy a drink now and then on the Snack Factor Diet by making a trade-off—just follow the guidelines I've explained in Chapter 6. And there's no reason not to. Researchers have linked moderate alcohol consumption (defined as one drink a day) with improved cardiovascular health, and even with a lower incidence of diabetes. Whenever you hoist a glass, though, you can still think about nutrient density: a glass of red wine, for instance, has powerful antioxidants, and not too many extra calories, like a fruity drink.

"What if I overeat? Do I skip eating the next day?"

Never skip a meal or force yourself to go hungry—that kind of penance-and-reward system just doesn't work.

Every time you "fall off the wagon," whether it's because you ate too much of a recommended food or ate a food that's not recommended at all, just record it and calmly move on. Every snack, every meal is a new page, a totally clean slate. And nobody is perfect.

This is a good time to revisit the black-and-white thinking that sabotages so many diets. It's so easy for us to say, "I blew it—not only did I have pizza instead of a salad, I had three pieces. I might as well keep eating like a maniac all weekend, and start over on Monday."

There's no reason to punish yourself like that. I know it's corny, but I sometimes ask clients to visualize the way babies learn to walk. When they fall down, do they lie there and kick and scream and decide they won't try again until Monday morning, or until January 1? Of course not. They fuss a little, then pull themselves back up and try again. The Snack Factor Diet involves the same process. This isn't the way you're used to eating, so you will screw up, probably more than a few times. That's okay.

"By the way, I hate using my food journal. Can I stop?"

Sorry, but no. In fact, I'll bet the very reason you hate it is exactly the reason you need to keep it up. Lots of people say, "I hardly eat anything out of the ordinary, and I'm still gaining (or just not losing) weight." But when people actually record what they eat, they often find they've been drastically underestimating their intake, according to a study published in the *New England Journal of Medicine*. And I know, it *is* embarrassing to write down all the weird and inexplicable ways we cheat. (Believe me, there is nothing I haven't seen on these food diaries, from "½ a container of Duncan Hines frosting with celery" to "nutrition bars dipped in peanut butter!")

Need more evidence? The study done at the University of Pennsylvania School of Medicine found that dieters who kept food journals lost more weight in the weeks in which they recorded their food the most accurately, and less in weeks where they were sloppier. I tell my clients daily: not only can I help you more, but you will help yourself more if you write it down. You get the point: no matter what you eat, *write it down.*

"How do I get back on track?"

Just start fresh, without any dramatic "one last hot-fudge sundae before I go back on my diet forever" behavior. Remember, I expect you to get offtrack sometimes. If it was easy to stay on the straight and narrow, you'd have lost the weight long before now. I remember reading a quote from a business mogul whose company once failed in a takeover bid. His response was so simple: "They won. We lost. Next." It's the same thing with overeating. Don't waste your energy thinking negative thoughts about what happened. Instead, put that energy into imagining how good you'll feel when you put that emotional tortilla-chip bender behind you by choosing a bowl of homemade vegetable soup and a nourishing piece of pork tenderloin at your next meal.

"I was so good all week, and I actually gained a few pounds. I'm so discouraged—why isn't this diet working for me?"

Sometimes, scales can be very misleading. If you were sticking to the plan all week, and if you were focusing on the four core components—portions, proportions, nutrient density, and your HQ—I bet you really did lose weight, even if the scale disagrees. That's because most of us don't have a fixed weight, but a fixed weight range. At any point over a one- or two-day period, the same woman might weigh 143 or 139 pounds. What happens when we diet is that we don't so much "lose three pounds" as we slide into a lower four-pound range. But when we focus too much on the scale, it's so easy to get upset and go "comfort" ourselves with food, sabotaging the solid progress we made that week (even if it wasn't measurable in terms of pounds and ounces).

My advice? First, get used to this. These apparent setbacks are common—weight loss almost never happens in a straight downward motion. And if you want to stay on the plan long term, you'll need to devise a strategy that helps you get through these tough days. That's why I stress that patience and consistency are the two most important tools you'll need.

Second, try as hard as you can to remember that food and emotions are not the same thing: we're trying to eat when we're hungry, not when we're ticked off at the bathroom scale. And finally, even though I've mostly encouraged you to use your food journal to record what you eat (which gives you plenty of freedom), in this case, it helps to write down a plan for what you'll eat today. That way, you can follow it without thinking. Do I believe sitting down at bedtime and mapping out every morsel of food you'll consume the next day is a fun way to live? Of course not. But on these emotional days, when you feel discouraged about what seems like your lack of progress, these food plans can be a safeguard. Go to pages 153–54 to see the Food Planner. And I bet by the following day you'll have noticed another sign that you're losing weight— a jacket zipping more easily, a dress slipping on more smoothly— and that will set your spirits right.

Remember: how you feel matters much more than any old number on the scale.

"I feel as if I could kill for some potato chips or a bagel. Am I going through carbohydrate withdrawal?"

No, carbs aren't addictive, any more than sugar is. You're probably just craving carbs because you're hungry. Check your food journals, and make sure you're hitting all the food groups. Make a sandwich with fiber crackers, or go for a heartier vegetable serving, such as squash, and see if that satisfies your craving. Finally, if all else fails, make one of those foods you're craving—in a calorically controlled portion—one of your conscious indulgences this week.

"I love popcorn, but the labels drive me nuts, with different calorie counts for what's popped and unpopped."

Me, too! That's why I suggest that my popcorn-loving clients keep it simple, and just buy the Jolly Time 100-Calorie microwave bags. Or for you air-popping people out there, 2 tablespoons makes 5 cups popped, or about 100 calories worth.

I sometimes do not need a yogurt and a fat. Can I split my snacks?

Absolutely! If you eat your healthy lunch and an hour later need a little something, maybe a Dannon Light & Fit Smoothie is perfect for you, but the 10 almonds may be too much at that moment and you push to a 3 on your HQ. You are better off having the yogurt drink and then later (maybe before going out to dinner) you can have the almonds and keep your HQ at a nice 4 to 6.

An Extra Helping

Six Keys to Overall Health

While eating well is incredibly important for good health, there are other factors involved in maintaining general wellness, a healthy weight, and high energy level. These are also things that keep us looking good and they keep us feeling even better. Who doesn't want to feel great and look great?

I talk about these other areas—exercise, fluids, stress management, sleep, and personal time–with all my clients and in all my work. Yes, it's true that I'm professionally trained as a registered dietitian, not as a shrink or a sleep expert. But I learned early on that no matter how focused a person is on losing weight, it's important to help the person keep an eye on the big picture. Total health and wellness and establishing lifestyle habits that will keep someone fit for decades are so much more important than what size jeans the person wears to an upcoming class reunion.

Often, people who have been working to lose weight have a black-and-white attitude that affects how they eat. Most of us are all too familiar with that "I had too much to eat Friday night—I may as well eat everything in sight until Monday morning" syndrome. Many people extend that kind of all-or-nothing mentality to other health decisions. Because they're not eating well, they seem to feel the need to punish themselves in other ways. They won't drink enough water, for example, or maybe even not take time out to see an old friend. I've had clients who refuse to exercise until they feel their eating is "back on track." This type of feast-or-famine roller-coaster living is incredibly unhealthy.

Since you've stuck with me right through to the final chapter, I know you're on board with an approach to eating that involves lots of dieting strategies, not just one or two. And within a few days, you probably got the hang of how watching your HQ, portions, proportions, and nutrient density offered you different tools for managing your hunger. Now I'm going to show you how paying attention to other important lifestyle issues will help you achieve your goal weight.

Sometimes, I get a little resistance from clients on this issue. They want to insist that their weight depends solely on what they eat or don't eat each day. But pretty quickly I can convince them that that is a very shortsighted way to view weight loss. Let's say you're finishing up a killer project at work, and it's added stress and cut into your sleep. Imagining that those changes aren't going to affect the way you eat— and even the way your body handles the calories you feed it— is just naive. Even if it doesn't affect you physiologically, it can affect you mentally, which in turn affects your eating. My clients tell me that when they adopt this balanced approach to life, it helps them feel happier, stronger, and more relaxed than they've ever felt before.

Will you be able to practice all six keys to overall health all the time? I doubt it. Most of us lead busy lives and are always struggling to keep things in balance in one area or another. But the trick is to keep trying to regain your balance after an upset, with patience and consistency. Soon, regrouping after a setback—whether it's a bad cold, a strained hamstring, or a doughnut binge–will get easier and easier. So you didn't sleep well last night and inhaled a box of cookies at your desk? That doesn't mean you still can't go to the gym after work, eat a great dinner, and then tuck yourself into bed early tonight after relaxing with the scent of lavender candles. As you gain a greater sense of balance, you'll get sick less often, and you'll discover a kind of steady self-reliance you didn't know you had. Also, you will never have to live through those jarring up-and-down, on-the-health-wagon-and-off, all-or-nothing cycles again.

DRINKING FLUIDS

As you've heard a thousand times, our bodies are 50 to 75 percent water, and we need to drink at least eight glasses a day to function at our best. Most people don't know that the most common reason people are sluggish in the afternoon is dehydration. If we don't drink enough water, our bodies do not function properly. We become tired and don't metabolize food properly. And we miss out on that clean, healthy, and refreshed feeling we get from drinking water.

I always tell clients to start their day with a warm glass of lemon water. That little blast of vitamin C is so healthy, and in Ayurvedic medicine, lemon juice in warm water is believed to cleanse and tone the liver, keeping it in greater health to metabolize the food we consume. It's also a great way to wake up your digestive system each morning.

Next, I recommend that clients drink a glass of water before and during each meal. Sometimes, they think I tell them this because water fills them up, and therefore they'll eat less. But that's really not the reason I suggest it, although it may do this for you, too! It's because drinking water at every meal is probably the single best way to make water a habit, not an afterthought. (And to some people, it's less of a nuisance than carting a full liter of Evian everywhere they go.) So even if these were the only two hydration tips of mine you follow, you're already drinking seven glasses a day.

Flavoring water with either lemon (I recommend True Lemon travel packets, which are easy to carry when you're on the go) or cucumbers (a refreshing trick from Asian countries) also makes it more appealing. And when clients are really craving diet soda, I suggest they try seltzer and add lemon or lime so they can get their bubbly fix.

Herbal teas are another great source. Take a tea break for green, black, white, or herbal tea midmorning and mid-afternoon. (But keep in mind that most green, black, and white teas do contain some caffeine.)

Finally, limit the amount of alcohol you consume. Not only does it dehydrate you, but sipping wine all evening tricks you into thinking you're not thirsty, when in fact your body is craving fluids. Choose the nights when you'll drink alcohol and cut drinks in half each night you drink, or incorporate one of your conscious indulgences.

MANAGING STRESS

Stress is just a normal part of life, and we need a certain amount of it to function. In normal situations, the body's physiological reaction to stress is simple: you're racing to make a 3:00 P.M. deadline, and your body kicks out enough adrenaline to get your heart pumping. Every part of your brain and body seems focused on getting this report done on time. Once the deadline passes, you relax, and your heart rate and blood chemicals return to normal levels.

The problems start when we are constantly under stress. Chronic stress causes elevated levels of cortisol, and over time, this is a drain on our immune system, making us more vulnerable to minor illnesses like colds, as well as major ones like cancer and heart disease. (By the way, cortisol isn't the only "bad" stress hormone, but it is the most abundant of the steroid hormones called glucocorticoids.)

Cortisol also makes our bodies crave carbohydrates—specifically high-sugar carbohydrates—and store fat around the midsection. So even if you don't eat more due to stress, you can still gain weight. (Sorry to tell you, but those diet aids you've seen advertised on late-night TV that claim to combat cortisol-related weight loss don't work.)

To make matters worse, stress also causes an increase in appetite. We all know what that does. For the many people who are known as emotional eaters—people who eat to calm their feelings—stress affects the foods they choose. A study from the University College in London involved stressing out half of a group of sixty-eight volunteers by telling them to prepare a speech that they would give after lunch, which would be videotaped and then critiqued. (I bet even reading that sentence made your palms sweat—public speaking is one of the most stressful events there is for most people.) It turns out that under stress, the "emotional eaters" ate more calories overall and especially more foods that were high in both sugar and fat.

Women seem to be especially vulnerable to the stress-overeating connection. A study at the University of Liverpool offered volunteers as much chocolate as they wanted after completing stressful tasks—and researchers found that women were more likely to overeat than men were.

So if stress is an amazing food trigger, what can you do about it? Plenty! Besides exercise (more on that in a minute), the most effective way to lower stress is through meditation. And no, I'm not expecting you to join an ashram to help lose weight. In terms of calming you down and starting what doctors have long called "the relaxation response," meditation can be anything from knitting, deep breathing, or simply sitting on your porch and watching the clouds drift by. Any soothing, rhythmic activity—for some people, that's running; for others, it can be playing the bagpipes—that causes you to breathe deeply is a surefire stress buster.

There are plenty of good tapes and CDs to get you started, and many yoga classes end with simple breathing meditations. You can even download plenty of free meditations online. Or if that's too complicated, just sit still for ten minutes a day, and don't do anything but breathe. Count ten slow, deep breaths, then start over. I also recommend lighting incense or a candle and doing this breathing for five minutes before bedtime.

Be prepared for powerful results. Doctors at Duke University have found that teaching patients with Type 2 diabetes such simple meditation techniques enabled them to lower their glucose levels—just by breathing!

SMART SLEEPING

When you are well rested, you make better food choices and have more energy to go the gym, walk to work, or take time for your favorite activities. When you are not well rested, your defenses are down and you are more likely to overeat and make poor food choices. You're more likely to feel moody, and if you are the kind of person who eats emotionally, you're setting yourself up for a diet disaster. And there's one more thing. Remember cortisol? Lack of sleep makes this hormone rise as well.

Researchers at the University of Chicago found that people who don't get enough sleep have an 18 percent decrease in leptin, the hormone that tells us when we're satisfied, and a 28 percent increase in ghrelin, the hormone that tells us we're hungry. So it's not surprising, then, that the people who volunteered for the study—and were restricted to four hours of sleep for two nights in a row—reported a 24 percent increase in appetite, with an especially strong desire for sweets, salty foods, and starches.

For people who are generally good sleepers, the solution is as simple as making a conscious decision to get the seven or eight hours they need each night. But for people who suffer from some level of sleep problems, either an occasional sleepless night or chronic insomnia, it can be much trickier. Exercising every day will help a great deal, as will eliminating caffeine. Turning off all electronics—yes, TV *and* your computer—a half hour or so before bedtime will also help. So will any soothing rituals you can think of: a hot bath, rubbing lotion on your hands, a few pages of a book, a little yoga, or listening to calming music.

EXERCISING OFTEN

Talk about a miracle cure! Aside from burning calories, exercise is an antidote to stress and a cure for some sleep problems. But regular exercise does so much *more* for our bodies. It releases endorphins, a cascade of hormones that just make us feel good! That sense of well-being motivates people to eat well, do their job well, and simply be happy.

In some ways, encouraging clients who used to exercise and have fallen out of the habit is easier (they are inspired by memories of what great shape they *used* to be in). It doesn't take many trips to the gym before they remember how much they liked to exercise, how they enjoyed that calm feeling of accomplishment when they finished, and how they started to crave exercise when a few days went by without it.

It's a little tougher to motivate someone who remembers high school gym as its own kind of torture and still has nightmares about dodgeball. And it's especially disconcerting for those who have read the U.S. surgeon general's latest guidelines on exercise, which recommend that anyone looking to lose weight exercise for ninety minutes at a time, most days of the week. "Ninety minutes?" I've had clients say. *"Ninety?!"*

"Relax," I tell them. "In the beginning, any amount of exercise is a great start." Strive for at least four sessions of exercise a week, but it's important to make realistic goals. Often, people say, "I'm going to exercise every day this week," and then they get discouraged when they don't follow through. Is seven times a week realistic? So ask yourself what suits your schedule this week—maybe two sessions during the week? Maybe two on the weekends?

There are three kinds of exercise, each of them very important:

- **Cardiovascular fitness.** This refers to the kind of exercise that cranks your heart rate up and protects you against heart disease. It also burns the most calories and is very beneficial in managing stress. Start by walking or running around the neighborhood for twenty minutes, and before long, you will find it easier to run for thirty or forty minutes.

    But daily activity also counts, so think of ways to work more activity into your everyday routines: cut the grass with a push mower, or trick yourself into going up and down stairs more often. I know that you've heard all these ideas before, but the idea is, with patience and consistency, to work them into your regular life. That's how they become habits.

- **Weight-bearing exercise.** If you don't belong to a gym, pick up some free weights at a sporting goods store because weights may turn out to be your most important weight-loss tool. Resistance training, which includes lifting free weights, working out on weight machines, and doing push-ups, increases lean muscle. That revs up the metabolism and increases the number of calories the body burns at rest. People who lift weights burn more calories than people who don't, even when they are just sitting on the couch. Researchers at the University of Maryland have found that the resting metabolic rate increased by about 7 percent after six months of intense weight training.

  Weight training is especially rewarding for people who are impatient. After even a few weeks, you'll start to notice better definition, as your body builds lean muscle. Bonus: weight training, which strengthens bones as well as muscles, is one of the best defenses against osteoporosis.

- **Flexibility.** This third component of fitness is often the easiest one for people to ignore. After all, it doesn't blast calories, like a stair-stepper, or perk up your butt, as weight training will. But flexibility is important because it prevents injuries and makes weight training work better. (People who stretch between sets build muscle more quickly than people who don't.) And besides, if done right, stretching feels *so* good. If you haven't already, experiment with a beginning yoga class, or at the very least, take ten minutes after each workout to cool down and stretch out your muscles.

And for those of you who are already consistent about your workout, but not happy with your weight, it's time to crank it up a little with intervals. Interval training can help rev your metabolism for hours, even after you have left the gym. On the bike or treadmill, try thirty seconds at your max, followed by two minutes at a more relaxed pace. Run or walk outdoors, sprint between every third telephone pole, or change your route to incorporate some hills. Continue with these intervals for at least ten minutes, one workout a week.

If you already lift weights, treat yourself to a session with a personal trainer. He or she can help you spot the bad habits most of us form, and help you add a few new moves to get better results.

And above all, try something new once in a while. People who grow bored with running the same four miles on the treadmill, day after day, year after year, are more likely to abandon exercising entirely. Sign up for a session of rock climbing, spend an afternoon ice skating, or take a tap dancing class.

MAKING TIME FOR YOURSELF

What good is all this working out, meditation, and sleeping if you have no time to enjoy your good health? Remember, you are a better friend, spouse, parent, boss, and employee when you are happy and feel good about *yourself.* Sometimes, my clients get so swept up in all the healthy things that I need to remind them that they should treat themselves to an afternoon of shopping, a stroll through a new art gallery, or a day at the driving range.

It's also important to remember to schedule downtime for yourself—those restorative hours when you read a good book, laze around the house, and maybe even take a Sunday afternoon nap. Your stress levels will go down, and you will be more motivated to live your best life.

EATING WELL

Obviously, eating well is about the most important thing you can do to take care of yourself. And as you get more familiar with the Snack Factor Diet, you'll start to think of it not just as a way to lose weight but also as part of who you are. In fact, the best thing is when my clients tell me, "This doesn't feel like a diet anymore. It feels as if I'm finally learning to take care of myself. It is so livable!"

NOTES

Great new products hit the market all the time, while others disappear. The field of nutrition is constantly evolving. Please check my Web site regularly for updates in research, standout products, new snacks, and useful tools (such as food journals and meal planners). And feel free to e-mail me with any questions at www.snackfactordiet.com

This chapter contains the references to specific studies I've mentioned in the book. If you want to learn more about the many studies I use in my practice (those not already mentioned here), I'd like to suggest two sources. The first is PubMed, a Web site overseen by the National Institutes of Health, which includes research from thousands of *academic* sources.

Just type "PubMed" into your favorite search engine, put in a key word, and you'll get many—sometimes hundreds!—of research articles related to topics I've addressed in this book.

Many universities have set up health-oriented Web sites that are also very user-friendly. One that I like is the Tufts University Health & Nutrition Letter. And I'm not just saying that because that's where I got my undergraduate degree. The Tufts Friedman School of Nutrition Science and Policy is one of the country's leading nutrition research institutions. Just go to healthletter.tufts.edu and enter a key word in the search field. Another great resource is Harvard University's health Web site, health.harvard.edu.

As far as the studies mentioned here, I've organized the notes this way: First, I give the phrase in the book chapter, followed by the title of the academic article, the authors, and then the abbreviated name of the scholarly journal. (They may look funny, but that's for ease of use—typing in the abbreviations will likely get you to a given study faster than taking the time to spell it out.) And if I'm citing information provided by a government or scientific agency, rather than academic research, I've given the Web address that should take you straight to the right page.

Introduction: Eat Up! It's Healthy

2 **But please understand that you're not alone: *60 percent of America is overweight:*** http://www.cdc.gov/nccdphp/publications/aag/dnpa.htm.

6 **A study from a medical school in South Africa measured it this way:** "Greater Appetite Control Associated with an Increased Frequency of Eating in Lean Males," D. P. Speechly and R. Buffenstein, *Appetite*, 33, no. 3 (1999):285–97.

6 **Another study tracked a group of French adults:** "Contribution of Snacks and Meals in the Diet of French Adults: A Diet-Diary Study," F. Bellisle, A. M. Dalix, L. Mennen, P. Galan, S. Hercberg, J. M. de Castro, and N. Gausseres, *Physiol Behav*, 79, no. 2 (2003):183–89.

7 **Studies found that when regular fourth-meal eaters gave up that afternoon snack:** "Highlighting the Positive Impact of Increasing Feeding Frequency on Metabolism and Weight Management," J. Louis-Sylvestre, A. Lluch, F. Neant, and J. E. Blundell, *Forum Nutr*, 56 (2003):126–28.

7 **One study tracked obese people:** "Reduced Stomach

Capacity in Obese Subjects after Dieting," A. Geliebter, S. Schachter, C. Lohmann-Walter, H. Feldman, and S. A. Hashim, *Am J Clin Nutr*, 63, no. 2 (1996): 170–73.

7   **A study of more than 3,200 men and women, conducted by Arizona State University:** "Snacking Patterns Influence Energy and Nutrient Intakes But Not Body Mass Index," J. S. Hampl, C. L. Heaton, and C. A. Taylor, *J Hum Nutr Diet*, 16, no. 1 (2003): 1–2.

8   **Research has also confirmed how snacking helps heart health. One clinical trial, for example:** "Regular Meal Frequency Creates More Appropriate Insulin Sensitivity and Lipid Profiles Compared with Irregular Meal Frequency in Healthy Lean Women," H. R. Farshchi, M. A. Taylor, I. A. Macdonald, *Eur J Clin Nutr*, 58, no. 7 (2004): 1071–77.

9   **Best of all, snacking makes us happier:** "The Influence of Breakfast and a Snack on Psychological Functioning," D. Benton, O. Slater, R. T. Donohoe, *Physiol Behav*, 74, no. 4–5 (2001): 559–71.

Chapter 1: What's Your H.Q.?

14   **The Pima Indians in the Southwest:** "Diabetes Mellitus in the Pima Indians: Genetic and Evolutionary Considerations," W. C. Knowler, D. J. Pettitt, P. H. Bennett, and R. C. Williams, *Am J Phys Anthropol* 62, no. 1 (1983): 107–14.

18   **Recently, researchers at the University of Pittsburgh learned that C-reactive protein:** "Induction of Leptin Resistance Through Direct Interaction of C-Reactive Protein with Leptin," K. Chen, F. Li, J. Li, H. Cai, S. Strom, A. Bisello, and D. Kelley, *Nat Med*, 12, no. 4 (2006): 425–32.

19   **Studies have shown that people in this category:** "Stress and Eating: The Effects of Ego-Threat and Cognitive Demand on Food Intake in Restrained and Emotional Eaters," D. J. Wallis, M. M. Hetherington, *Appetite*, 43, no. 1 (2004): 39–46.

21   **A group of healthy-weight women were given the same**

number of calories per day: "Decreased Thermic Effect of Food After an Irregular Compared with a Regular Meal Pattern in Healthy Lean Women," H. R. Farshchi, M. A. Taylor, and I. A. Macdonald, *Int J Obes Relat Metab Disord*, 28, no. 5 (2004): 653–60.

Chapter 2: Thinking in Thirds

30 **Between 1991, just before the USDA introduced the Food Pyramid, and 2000**: http://www.cdc.gov/od/oc/media/pressrel/r010911.htm.

31 **In reality, a typical Atkins-type day provided:** http://www.atkinsdietalert.org/advisory.html.

32 **The Women's Health Initiative released a massive study that showed that low-fat diets didn't provide many of the health benefits:** http://www.whi.org/findings/dm/dm.php.

35 **Researchers at the University of Washington in Seattle recently took a group:** "High-Protein Diet, Obesity, and the Environment," F. Contaldo and F. Pasanisi. *Am J Clin Nutr*, 83, no. 2 (2006): 387.

36 **One Harvard University study looked at more than 900 cases of heart disease in women:** "Dietary Protein and Risk of Ischemic Heart Disease in Women," F. Hu, M. Stamper, J. Manson, E. Rimm, G. Colditz, F. Speizer, C. Hennekens, and W. Willett, *Am J Clin Nutr*, 70, no. 2 (1999): 221–27.

36 **An analysis from a group of researchers in the Netherlands determined that moderate-protein diets:** "High Protein Intake Sustains Weight Maintenance After Body Weight Loss in Humans," M. S. Westerterp-Plantenga, M. P. G. M. Lejeune, I. Nijs, M. van Ooijen and E. M. R. Kovacs, *Int J Obes*, 28, (2004): 57–64.

36 **At the Harvard School of Public Health, researchers recently sifted through more than fifty previously published studies:** "The Effects of High Protein Diets on Thermogenesis, Satiety and Weight Loss: A Critical Review," T. Halton and F. Hu, *J Am Coll Nutr*, 23, no. 5 (2004): 373–85.

39   **But there's an added bonus because lean proteins provide an extra boost to satiety levels:** "A Comparison of Effects of Fish and Beef Protein on Satiety in Normal Weight Men," S. Borzoei, *Eur J Clin Nutr*, 60, no. 7 (2006): 897–902.

39   **But a recent study did find that 6 percent of the chunk light sampled contained the same level of mercury or higher than white:** http://fsnep.ucdavis.edu/ffc/press/ pressmain.cfm?type=style&ffcrelease=ffcpress0000003.cfm.

42   **Many studies have shown that of the three groups:** "The Satiating Power of Protein—A Key to Obesity Prevention?" A. Astrup, *Am J Clin Nutr*, 82, no. 1 (2005): 1–2. Another study: "Fat as a Risk Factor for Overconsumption: Satiation, Satiety, and Patterns of Eating," J. E. Blundell, and J. MacDiarmid, *J Am Diet Assoc*, 97, no. 7 (1997): S63–169.

43   **British researchers have found that as the rate at which the stomach empties changes, so does its hormonal response to food:** "Fats and Food Intake," S. French and T. Robinson, *Curr Opin Clin Nutr Metab Care*, 6, no. 6 (2003): 629–34.

43   **Researchers have shown that when rats are given the chance to choose such foods:** "Dietary-Induced Overeating in Experimental Animals," R. B. Kanarek and E. Hirsch. *Fed Proc*, 36, no.2 (1997): 154–58.

44   **The longer-chain omega-6 fats are commonly found in vegetable oils:** Enter "IOM 2002 Report, Dietary Reference Intakes for Energy, Carbohydrate, Fiber, Fat, Fatty Acids, Cholesterol, Protein, and Amino Acids" into a search engine, click on the PDF file, and you'll find this information on page 4.

44   **A recent study published in the *American Journal of Clinical Nutrition* showed that salads with "regular" salad dressing:** "Carotenoid Bioavailability is Higher from Salads Ingested with Full Fat Than with Fat-Reduced Salad Dressings as Measured with Electrochemical Detection," M. J. Brown, M. G. Ferruzzi, M. L. Nguyen, D. A. Cooper, A. L. Elrdige, S. J. Schwartz, and W. S. White, *Am J Clin Nutr*, 80 (2004): 396–403.

44 **A word of caution, though: at Harvard Medical School, researchers have found that when people are already suffering from angina or congestive heart failure, omega-3s may increase the risk of cardiac death:** "Blood Levels of Long-Chain n–3 Fatty Acids and the Risk of Sudden Death," C. M. Albert, H. Campos, M. J. Stampfer, P. M. Ridker, J. E. Manson, W. C. Willett, and J. Ma, *N Engl J Med*, 346 (2002):1113–18.

45 **These heighten the risk of heart disease in some people by boosting the level of harmful, low-density lipoprotein cholesterol in the bloodstream:** "Trans Fatty Acids and Cardiovascular Disease," D. Mozaffarian, M. B. Katan, A. Ascherio, M. J. Stampfer, and W. C. Willett, *N Engl J Med*, 354, no. 15 (2006): 1601–13.

45 **Researchers in Australia recently gave subjects a very high-fat breakfast:** "The Influence of the Type of Dietary Fat on Postprandial Fat Oxidation Rates: Monounsaturated (Olive Oil) vs Saturated Fat (Cream)," L. S. Piers, K. Z. Walker, R. M. Stoney, M. J. Soares, and K. O'Dea, *Int J Obes Relat Metab Disord*, 26, no.6 (2002): 8.

Chapter 3: Secrets of the Nutrient Bargain Hunter

49 **While those numbers are important to nutritionists, as well as to people with diabetes and prediabetes, I tell my clients not to pay too much attention:** If you'd like to learn more about the glycemic index, here's a good overvew from a leading source on diabetes: http://www.joslin.org/managing_your_diabetes_698.asp.

50 **Doctors are so bullish on fiber's ability to help control blood sugar levels that they recommend that people with diabetes eat even more fiber than the rest of us—up to 50 grams per day:** http://www.diabetesmonitor.com/m27.htm.

50 **Compared to the overall recommendations of 20 to 35 grams (38 grams for men ages 14–50) for other adults:** http://www.nlm.nih.gov/medlineplus/ency/article/002470.htm.

51   If you want the nitty-gritty details, scientists believe that
      there are several reasons why high-fiber foods score so
      well in satiety: "Dietary Fiber and Body Weight," J. L.
      Slavin, *Nutrition*, 21, no. 3 (2005): 411–18.

51   This seems especially important at breakfast. Studies
      have found that the higher the fiber content of breakfast,
      the less food we take in later in the day: "The Effect of
      Breakfast Type on Total Daily Energy Intake and Body Mass
      Index: Results from the Third National Health and Nutrition
      Examination Survey," S. Cho, M. Dietrich, C. J. P. Brown,
      C. A. Clark, and G. Block, *J Am Coll Nutr*, 22, no. 4 (2003):
      296–302.

56   Whole grains also seem to be essential to healthy weight
      loss. In the famous Harvard Nurse's Study, researchers
      found that the more high-fiber: "Relation Between Changes
      in Intakes of Dietary Fiber and Grain Products and Changes
      in Weight and Development of Obesity Among Middle-Aged
      Women," S. Liu, W. C. Willett, J. E. Manson, F. B. Hu, B.
      Rosner, and G. Colditz, *Am J Clin Nutr*, 78, no. 5 (2003):
      920–27.

58   Most scientists agree that babies are born with the in-
      stinctive preference for sweets: "Development of Food
      Preferences," L. L. Birch, *Annu Rev Nutr*, 19, (1999): 41–62.

59   Researchers agree that, unlike other established addic-
      tive substances, sugar does not cause uncontrollable
      cravings or lead to clinical withdrawal symptoms: http://
      www.rps.psu.edu/probing/sugar.html.

59   A study on rats at Princeton University showed the possible
      existence of a sugar "dependency": http://www.princeton.
      edu/pr/news/02/q2/0620-hoebel.htm.

61   Protein also has the most nutritional staying power.
      While the effect of simple carbs begins to wear off in
      thirty minutes or so: "Effects of Macronutrient Content and
      Energy Density of Snacks Consumed in a Satiety State on the
      Onset of the Next Meal," C. Marmonier, D. Chapelot, and
      J. Louis-Sylvestre, *Appetite*, 34, no. 2 (2002):161–68.

61   **Researchers at Saint Louis University found that women who started their day with an egg:** "Short-term Effect of Eggs on Satiety in Overweight and Obese Subjects," J. S. Vander Wal, J. M. Marth, P. Khosla, K. L. Jen, and N. V. Dhurandhar, *J Am Coll Nutr*, 24, no. 6 (2005): 510–15.

63   **They include essential fatty acids, monounsaturated fats, and polyunsaturated fats:** http://www.hsph.harvard.edu/nutritionsource/fats.html.

67   **The problem with these foods:** "How Palatable Food Disrupts Appetite Regulation," C. Erlanson-Albertsson, *Basic Clin Pharmacol Toxicol*, 97, no. 2 (2005): 61–73.

Chapter 4: How Much Can You Eat?

96   **Restaurant portions have gotten so out of control that the Food and Drug Administration is asking restaurants:** http://www.fda.gov/bbs/topics/NEWS/2006/NEW01379.html.

104   **Cinnamon is a wonderful addition to yogurt or cottage cheese, and also has potential health benefits:** "Effects of a Cinnamon Extract on Plasma Glucose, HbA, and Serum Lipids in Diabetes Mellitus Type 2," B. Mang, M. Wolters, R. Schmitt, K. Kelb, R. Lichtinghagen, D. O. Stichtenoth, and A. Hahn, *Eur J Clin Invest*, 36, no. 5 (2006): 340–44.

Chapter 5: The Snack Factor Diet

113   **No more excuses. Researchers have figured out that the dieters who *eat* breakfast lose significantly more weight over a twelve-week period than those who skip breakfast:** "The Role of Breakfast in the Treatment of Obesity: A Randomized Clinical Trial," D. G, Schlundt, J. O. Hill, T. Sbrocco, J. Pope-Cordle, and T. Sharp, *Am J Clin Nutr*, 55 (1992): 645–51.

113   **If you're still not convinced:** "Long-term Weight Loss and Breakfast in Subjects in the National Weight Control Registry," H. R. Wyatt, G. K. Grunwald, C. L. Mosca, M. L.

Klem, R. R. Wing, and J. O. Hill, *Obesity Research*, 10 (2002): 78–82.

112 **researchers know that snacks consumed when you're not hungry can make you gain weight:** "Snacks Consumed in a Nonhungry State Have Poor Satiating Efficiency: Influence of Snack Composition on Substrate Utilization and Hunger," C. Marmonier, D. Chapelot, M. Fantino, and S. Louis, *Am J Clin Nutr*, 76, no. 3 (2002): 518–28.

116 **Researchers have found that wild greens are a richer source of nutrients:** "Identification and Quantitation of Major Carotenoids in Selected Components of the Mediterranean Diet: Green Leafy Vegetables, Figs and Olive Oil," Q. Su, K. G. Rowley, C. Itsiopoulos, and K. O'Dea, *Eur J Clin Nutr*, 56, no. 11 (2002): 1149–54.

127 **Calcium's role in helping us lose weight is unclear. Researchers from the University of Tennessee:** "Calcium and Dairy Acceleration of Weight and Fat Loss During Energy Restriction in Obese Adults," M. B. Zemel, W. Thompson, A. Milstead, K. Morris, and P. Campbell, *Obes Res*, 12 (2004): 582–90.

127 **But a study from the prestigious Mayo Clinic in 2005:** "Effect of Energy-Reduced Diets High in Dairy Products and Fiber on Weight Loss in Obese Adults," W. G. Thompson, N. R. Holdman, D. J. Janzow, J. M. Slezak, K. L. Morris, and M. B. Zemel, *Obes Res*, 13, no. 8 (2005): 1344–53.

127 **But we do *know* that calcium protects bones. Osteoporosis:** Learn more about this problem at the Natrional Osteoporosis Foundation, http://www.nof.org/.

Chapter 6: Conscious Indulgences

158 **The average American goes to a restaurant 3.2 times per week, according to *Zagat:*** http://www.hotel-online.com/News/PR2004_4th/Nov04_Zagat.html.

Chapter 7: Troubleshooting

195 **And—as tedious as it is—there's plenty of evidence that the more slowly you shed those extra pounds, the more likely they are to stay gone:** "Whittling Away at Obesity and Overweight. Small Lifestyle Changes Can Have the Biggest Impact," C. B. Ruser, D. G. Federman, and S. S. Kashaf, *Postgrad Med*, 117, no. 1 (2005): 31–34, 37–40.

196 **nearly 600 men and women for a year, and found that most people do vary their diet and exercise habits by season, eating an average of 86 calories per day more in the fall than during the spring:** "Seasonal Variation in Food Intake, Physical Activity, and Body Weight in a Predominantly Overweight Population," Y. Ma, B. C. Olendzki, W. Li, A. R. Hafner, D. Chiriboga, J. R. Hebert, M. Campbell, M. Sarnie, I. S. Ockene, *Eur J Clin Nutr*, 60, no. 4 (2006): 519–28.

197 **One way to guard against those shifts, experts say, is to let seasonal changes naturally influence our diets:** "The Evolution of Human Fatness and Susceptibility to Obesity: An Ethological Approach," J. C. Wells, *Biol Rev Camb Philos Soc*, 1 (2006): 1–23.

197 **In a study by the Center for Behavioral Medicine in Chicago, groups of overweight people were divided into two groups:** "How Can Obese Weight Controllers Minimize Weight Gain During the High Risk Holiday Season? By Self-Monitoring Very Consistently." K. N. Boutelle, D. S. Kirschenbaum, R. C. Baker, and M. E. Mitchell, *Health Psychol*, 18, no. 4 (1999): 364–68.

202 **But when people actually record what they eat, they often find they've been drastically underestimating their intake, according to a study published in the *New England Journal of Medicine*:** "Randomized Trial of Lifestyle Modification and Pharmacotherapy for Obesity," T. A. Wadden, R. I. Berkowitz, L. G. Womble, D. B. Sarwer, S. Phelan, R. K. Cato, L. A. Hesson, S. Y. Osei, R. Kaplan, and A. J. Stunkard, *N Engl J Med*, 353, no. 20 (2005): 2111–20.

Chapter 8: An Extra Helping

210 **A study from the University College in London involved stressing out half of a group of sixty-eight volunteers by telling them:** "Stress and Food Choice: A Laboratory Study," G. Oliver, J. Wardle, and E. L. Gibson, *Psychosom Med*, 62, no. 6 (2002): 853–65.

211 **Be prepared for powerful results. Doctors at Duke University have found that:** "Stress Management Improves Long-term Glycemic Control in Type 2 Diabetes," R. S. Surwit, M. A. van Tilburg, N. Zucker, C. C. McCaskill, P. Parekh, M. N. Feinglos, C. L. Edwards, P. Williams, and J. D. Lane, *Diabetes Care*, 25, no. 1 (2002): 30–34.

212 **Researchers at the University of Chicago found that people who don't get enough sleep:** http://www.uchospitals. edu/news/2004/20041206-sleep.html.

213 **And it's especially disconcerting for those who have read the U.S. surgeon general's latest guidelines on exercise:** http://www.hhs.gov/news/press/2005pres/20050112.html.

214 **Researchers at the University of Maryland have found that the resting metabolic rate increased:** "Effect of Strength Training on Resting Metabolic Rate and Physical Activity: Age and Gender Comparison." J. T. Lemmer, F. M. Ivey, A. S. Ryan, G. F. Martel, D. E. Hurlbut, J. E. Metter, J. L. Fozard, J. L. Fleg, and B. F. Hurley, *Med Sci Sports Exerc*, 33, no. 4 (2001): 532–41.

APPENDIX

MUST-HAVES FROM THE GROCERY STORE

This list is meant to help you keep your pantry stocked even in its most basic form. This way you always have something to help you create a perfect meal using the Snack Factor chart. Using the portions list in Chapter 4, you can build a more elaborate grocery list.

STARCH
Cereal: Kellogg's All-Bran Extra Fiber
Oatmeal packets: Uncle Sam
Crackers: GG Scandinavian Bran Crispbread
Whole-grain bread: Arnold Bakery Light 100% Whole Wheat

MILK/YOGURT
Cottage cheese: Light & Lively Low-Fat
Low-fat cheese: Alpine Lace or Laughing Cow Light
Skim or soy milk: Skim Plus or Silk Soy
Yogurt: FAGE Total 0%

FRUIT AND VEGETABLES

Frozen
Vegetables: Cascadian Farms

Fresh
Apples
Baby carrots
Bagged lettuce
Blueberries
Celery
Cucumbers
Grapefruit
Grape tomatoes
Lemons
Spinach

MEAT OR MEAT SUBSTITUTE
Eggs: Eggology 100% Egg Whites, Country Hen Organic Eggs with Omega-3's
Tuna: Starkist vacuum-packed packages
Fish: EcoFish or other frozen wild salmon
Meat: Lean ground turkey
Veggie burgers: Dr. Praeger California Burger or Gardenburger

FAT
Natural peanut butter: Arrowhead Mills
Nuts: almonds, peanuts, walnuts

DRINKS
Green tea
Herbal teas

CONDIMENTS

Balsamic vinegar

Olive oil

TrueLemon packets

Mustard

Salt and pepper

FOOD STORAGE SUPPLIES

Ziploc snack-size zipper bags

Don't forget to ask your local grocery store or health food store to buy the products you cannot find. You would be surprised how often stores will respond to these requests.

FOOD JOURNAL

Date:	MONDAY	TUESDAY	WEDNESDAY	THURSDAY	FRIDAY	SATURDAY	SUNDAY
Exercise: Water							
Breakfast: Time: HQ: Mood:							
Snack: Time: HQ: Mood:							
Lunch: Time: HQ: Mood:							
Snack: Time: HQ: Mood:							
Dinner: Time: HQ: Mood:							

FOOD JOURNAL

Date:	MONDAY	TUESDAY	WEDNESDAY	THURSDAY	FRIDAY	SATURDAY	SUNDAY
Exercise: Water							
Breakfast: Time: HQ: Mood							
Snack: Time: HQ: Mood:							
Lunch: Time: HQ: Mood:							
Snack: Time: HQ: Mood:							
Dinner: Time: HQ: Mood:							

FOOD PLANNER

A food planner is different from a food journal in that the food planner helps you to map out your week ahead. It is especially useful when you know you have social engagements, are very busy, or are going to be home to cook. It can also help you to plan your shopping and your conscious indulgences.

Sample Day:	MONDAY	TUESDAY	WEDNESDAY	THURSDAY	FRIDAY	SATURDAY	SUNDAY
Breakfast Oatmeal Pancake							
Snack Asparagus spears							
Lunch Lite Cobb Salad							
Snack KeriBar							
Dinner (Out to dinner for friend's birthday: 1 glass of wine)							

RESOURCES

Great nutrition databases to look up food information:

www.eatright.org

www.intelihealth.com

www.mayoclinic.com

www.mrsgreens.com

www.NIH.gov

www.vitalchoice.com

www.webMD.com

www.whfoods.com

www.wholefoods.com

www.wildoats.com

INDEX